Pocket Atlas of Sectional Anatomy
Volume 1

Pocket Atlas of Sectional Anatomy

Computed Tomography and Magnetic Resonance Imaging

Volume 1
Head, Neck, Spine, and Joints

Torsten B. Moeller, M.D.
Am Caritas-Krankenhaus
Dillingen/Saar
Germany

Emil Reif, M.D.
Am Caritas-Krankenhaus
Dillingen/Saar
Germany

Second Edition, Revised and Expanded

318 Illustrations

Thieme
Stuttgart · New York 2000

Library of Congress Cataloging-in-Publication Data

Moeller, Torsten B.
  [Taschenatlas der Schnittbildanatomie. English]
  Pocket atlas of sectional anatomy, computed tomography and magnetic resonance imaging /
  Torsten B. Moeller, Emil Reif ; [translated by T. Telger]. – 2nd ed.
    p. ; cm
  Rev. ed. of: Pocket atlas of cross-sectional anatomy. 1994.
  Includes bibliographical references and index.
  Contents: v. 1. Head, neck, spine and joints – v. 2. Thorax, abdomen, and pelvis.
  ISBN 3 13 1255021 (GTV) – ISBN 0-86577-813-2 (TNY)
  1. Human anatomy-Atlases. 2. Tomography-Atlases. 3. Magnetic resonance imaging-Atlases. I. Reif,
  Emil. E, Moeller, Torsten B. Pocket atlas of sectional anatomy. III. Title.
  [DNLM: 1. Anatomy, Regional, Atlases. 2. Magnetic Resonance Imaging-Atlases. 3. Tomography,
  X-Ray Computed-Atlases. QS 17 M726t 2000a]
  QM25 M55513 2000
  611'.9'0222–dc21
                                               99-462369

Translated by T. Telger, Ft. Worth, TX, USA

This book is an authorized and revised translation of the 2nd German edition published and copyrighted 1997 by Georg Thieme Verlag, Stuttgart, Germany. Title of the German edition: Taschenatlas der Schnittbildanatomie

1st German edition 1993
1st English edition 1994
2nd German edition 1997

Important Note: Medicine is an ever-changing science undergoing continual development. Research and clinical experience are continually expanding our knowledge, in particular our knowledge of proper treatment and drug therapy. Insofar as this book mentions any dosage or application, readers may rest assured that the authors, editors, and publishers have made every effort to ensure that such references are in accordance with *the state of knowledge at the time of production of the book.*

Nevertheless, this does not involve, imply, or express any guarantee or responsibility on the part of the publishers in respect to any dosage instructions and forms of application stated in the book. *Every user is requested to examine carefully* the manufacturer's leaflets accompanying each drug and to check, if necessary in consultation with a physician or specialist, whether the dosage schedules mentioned therein or the contraindications stated by the manufacturers differ from the statements made in the present book. Such examination is particularly important with drugs that are either rarely used or have been newly released on the market. Every dosage schedule or every form of application used is entirely at the user's own risk and responsibility. The authors and publishers request every user to report to the publishers any discrepancies or inaccuracies noticed.

© 1994, 2000 Georg Thieme Verlag,
Rüdigerstrasse 14, D-70469 Stuttgart,
Germany
Thieme New York, 333 Seventh Avenue,
New York, NY 10001, USA

Typesetting by primustype R. Hurler GmbH,
73274 Notzingen, Germany
typeset on Textline/HerculesPro
Printed in Germany by
Druckerei Grammlich, Pliezhausen

ISBN 3-13-125502-1 (GTV)
ISBN 0-86577-813-2 (TNY)   2   3   4   5

Dedicated to our parents,
Alfred and Friedel Moeller,
Dr. Emil and Edith Reif,
in love and gratitude

Preface to the First Edition

This book presents the basic anatomy needed to interpret modern sectional images.

In making a diagnosis from sectional images, even experienced diagnosticians must adapt their thinking to the sectional portrayal of anatomic features. The *Pocket Atlas of Sectional Anatomy* aims to facilitate this process by presenting the two modalities that have the greatest practical importance in modern sectional imaging—computed tomography and magnetic resonance imaging.

The importance of these modalities rests partly on their high resolution. We have therefore attempted to provide vivid, comprehensive coverage of sectional anatomic details while still making the book compact and easy to use. The four-color illustrations were considered an essential part of this goal.

The contents of the two volumes, which comprise a unit, follow a strict format in which each CT or MR image is accompanied by a correlative color diagram and a reduced-scale schematic drawing indicating the level of the section. This format conveys maximum information in a minimum of space.

All the images were obtained in patients or volunteers. We thank our radiological technologists, especially Michaela Knittel, Pia Saar, Gisela Wagner, Monjuri Paul, and Andrea Britz, for the many ways in which they helped with this book. The manuscript was typed by Helga Brettschneider and Gabi Müller. We express special thanks to Dr. Markus Bach, Dr. Patrick Rosar, and especially Dr. Beate Hilpert for reading the manuscript and making helpful suggestions.

Dillingen, September 1993 *Torsten B. Moeller, Emil Reif*

Preface to the Second Edition

Sectional anatomy in humans is unchanging, but medicine is in a state of flux—particularly with regard to diagnostic imaging. This fact has made it imperative to create a second edition of the *Pocket Atlas of Sectional Anatomy*. Thus, the sections on arterial and venous MR angiography have been completely revised and original illustrations have been replaced with new ones based on a 512 image matrix. We were very pleased with the voluminous and consistently positive correspondence, including valuable suggestions, that we received in response to the first edition. One result of this has been the inclusion of coronal cranial CT images for the head and neck specialty. We are still seeking to improve our book and would welcome any further criticisms and suggestions.

Dillingen, Fall 1999   *Torsten B. Moeller, Emil Reif*

Table of Contents

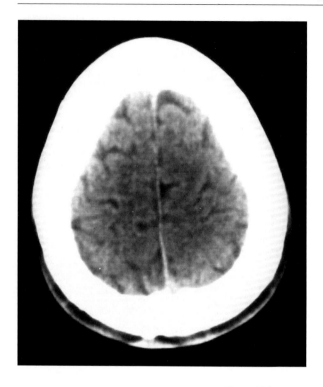

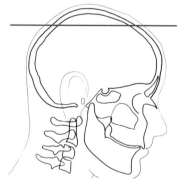

■ Frontal lobe
■ Parietal lobe

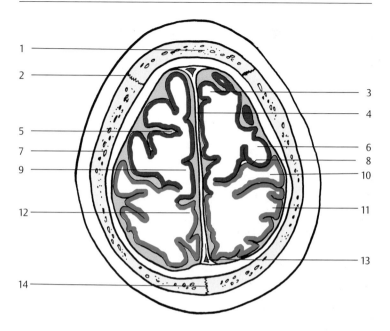

1 Frontal bone
2 Coronal suture
3 Superior frontal gyrus
4 Falx cerebri
5 Precentral sulcus
6 Precentral gyrus
7 Parietal bone

8 Central sulcus
9 Paracentral lobule
10 Postcentral gyrus
11 Superior parietal lobule
12 Precuneus
13 Superior sagittal sinus
14 Sagittal suture

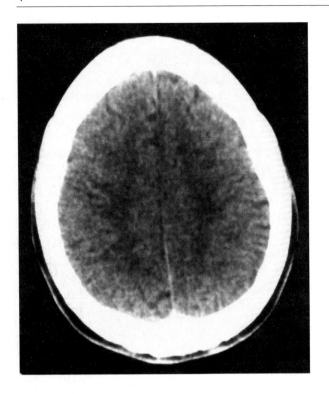

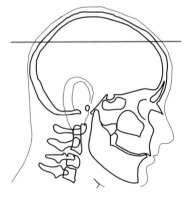

■ Frontal lobe
■ Parietal lobe

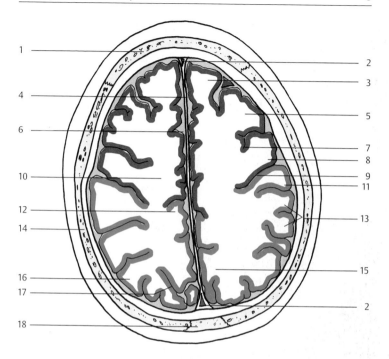

1   Frontal bone
2   Superior sagittal sinus
3   Superior frontal gyrus
4   Falx cerebri
5   Middle frontal gyrus
6   Longitudinal fissure
7   Precentral sulcus
8   Precentral gyrus
9   Central sulcus
10 Cerebral white matter
11 Postcentral gyrus
12 Paracentral lobule
13 Supramarginal gyrus
14 Parietal bone
15 Precuneus
16 Inferior parietal lobule
17 Parietooccipital sulcus
18 Occipital bone

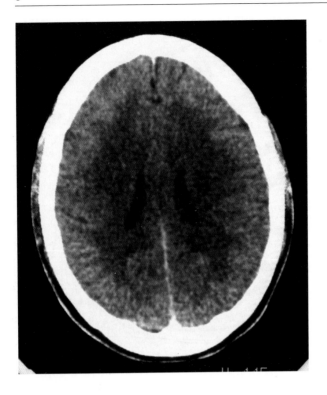

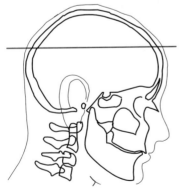

■ Frontal lobe
■ Parietal lobe
■ Occipital lobe

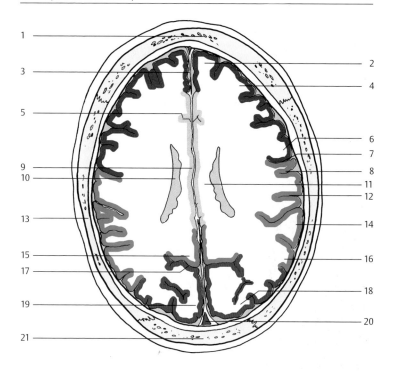

1 Frontal bone
2 Superior frontal gyrus
3 Falx cerebri
4 Middle frontal gyrus
5 Cingulate sulcus
6 Precentral gyrus
7 Central sulcus
8 Postcentral gyrus
9 Cingulate gyrus
10 Lateral ventricle (central part)
11 Cingulum

12 Postcentral sulcus
13 Parietal bone
14 Supramarginal gyrus
15 Precuneus
16 Angular gyrus
17 Parietooccipital sulcus
18 Occipital gyri
19 Cuneus
20 Superior sagittal sinus
21 Occipital bone

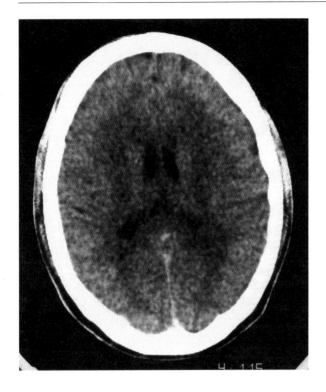

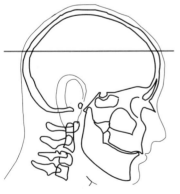

■ Frontal lobe
☐ Temporal lobe
■ Parietal lobe
■ Occipital lobe

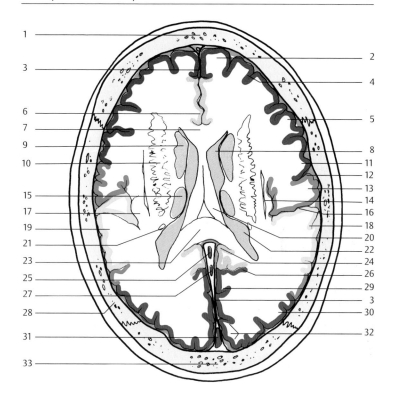

1 Frontal bone
2 Superior frontal gyrus
3 Falx cerebri
4 Middle frontal gyrus
5 Inferior frontal gyrus
6 Cingulate gyrus
7 Corpus callosum (trunk)
8 Lateral ventricle (anterior horn)
9 Caudate nucleus (head)
10 Corona radiata
11 Precentral gyrus
12 Central sulcus
13 Postcentral gyrus
14 Claustrum
15 Thalamus
16 Lateral sulcus
17 Insula
18 Superior temporal gyrus
19 Temporal operculum
20 Fornix
21 Caudate nucleus (tail)
22 Lateral ventricle (trigone, choroid plexus)
23 Corpus callosum (splenium)
24 Cingulum
25 Great cerebral vein
26 Parietooccipital sulcus
27 Straight sinus
28 Parietal bone
29 Cuneus
30 Occipital gyri
31 Superior sagittal sinus
32 Striate cortex
33 Occipital bone

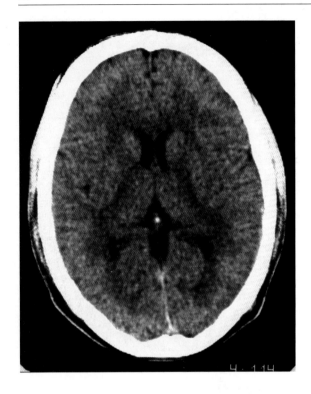

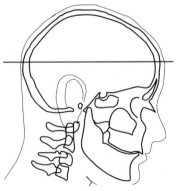

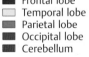

■ Frontal lobe
□ Temporal lobe
■ Parietal lobe
■ Occipital lobe
■ Cerebellum

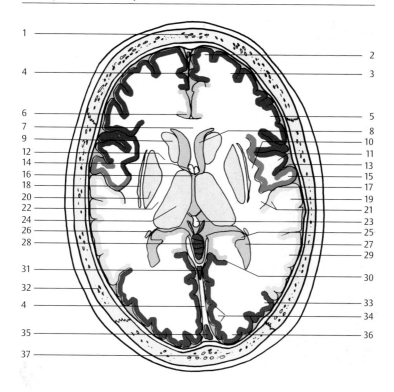

1 Frontal bone
2 Superior frontal gyrus
3 Middle frontal gyrus
4 Falx cerebri
5 Inferior frontal gyrus
6 Cingulate gyrus
7 Corpus callosum
8 Lateral ventricle (anterior horn)
9 Caudate nucleus (head)
10 Insula
11 Precentral gyrus
12 Internal capsule (anterior limb)
13 Central sulcus
14 Fornix
15 Postcentral gyrus
16 Interventricular foramen (of Monro)
17 Lateral sulcus
18 Claustrum
19 Superior temporal gyrus

20 Putamen
21 Transverse temporal gyrus
   (Heschl's gyrus)
22 Internal capsule (posterior limb)
23 Pineal gland
24 Thalamus
25 Hippocampus
26 Caudate nucleus (tail)
27 Lateral ventricle (trigone)
28 Vermis of cerebellum
29 Middle temporal gyrus
30 Parietooccipital sulcus
31 Straight sinus
32 Parietal bone
33 Occipital gyri
34 Striate cortex
35 Superior sagittal sinus
36 Occipital pole
37 Occipital bone

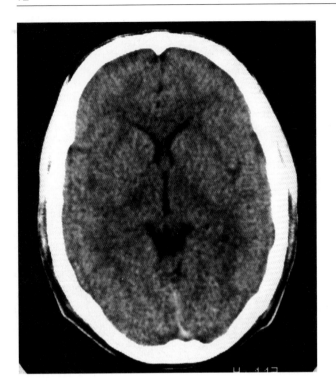

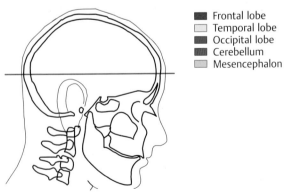

■ Frontal lobe
□ Temporal lobe
■ Occipital lobe
▤ Cerebellum
▦ Mesencephalon

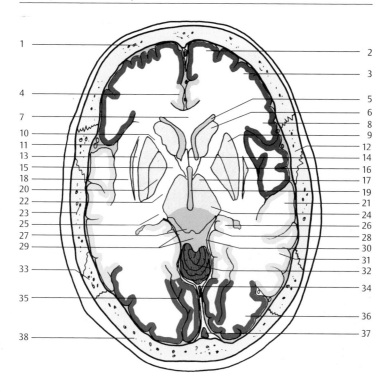

1 Frontal bone
2 Superior frontal gyrus
3 Middle frontal gyrus
4 Cingulate gyrus
5 Lateral ventricle (anterior horn)
6 Caudate nucleus (head)
7 Corpus callosum (genu)
8 Inferior frontal gyrus
9 Putamen
10 Internal capsule (anterior limb)
11 Insular cistern
12 Parietal bone
13 External capsule
14 Precommissural septum
15 Internal capsule (genu)
16 Claustrum
17 Hypothalamus
18 Capsula extrema
19 Third ventricle
20 Globus pallidus
21 Superior temporal gyrus
22 Internal capsule (posterior limb)
23 Temporal bone
24 Thalamus
25 Geniculate body
26 Hippocampus
27 Quadrigeminal plate (colliculus)
28 Parahippocampal gyrus
29 Quadrigeminal and ambient
   cisterns
30 Tentorium of cerebellum
31 Middle temporal gyrus
32 Vermis of cerebellum
33 Parietal bone
34 Straight sinus
35 Collateral sulcus
36 Occipital gyri
37 Superior sagittal sinus
38 Occipital bone

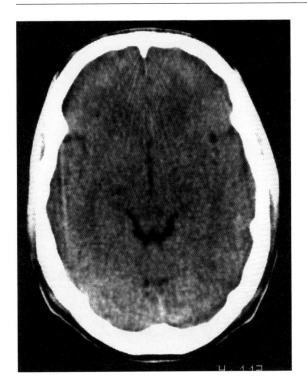

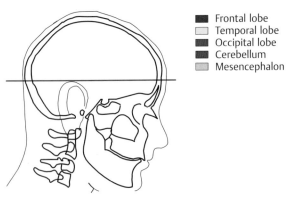

■ Frontal lobe
☐ Temporal lobe
▨ Occipital lobe
▩ Cerebellum
▦ Mesencephalon

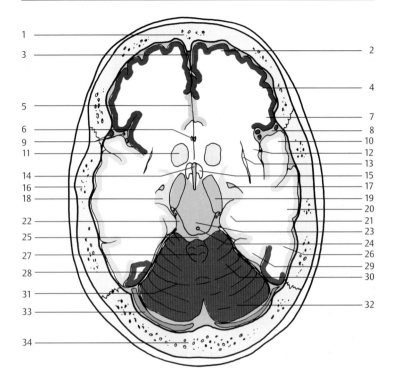

1 Frontal bone
2 Superior frontal gyrus
3 Falx cerebri
4 Middle frontal gyrus
5 Cingulate gyrus
6 Anterior cerebral artery
7 Inferior frontal gyrus
8 Lateral sulcus (insular cistern)
9 Insular arteries
10 Superior temporal gyrus
11 Corpus striatum (inferior portion)
12 Insula
13 Claustrum
14 Third ventricle
15 Hypothalamus
16 Parietal bone
17 Lateral ventricle (temporal horn)
18 Uncus

19 Cerebral peduncle
20 Middle temporal gyrus
21 Parahippocampal gyrus
22 Ambient cistern
23 Mesencephalon
24 Aqueduct
25 Quadrigeminal cistern
26 Inferior temporal gyrus
27 Vermis of cerebellum (superior portion)
28 Tentorium of cerebellum
29 Lateral occipitotemporal gyrus
30 Cerebellum (cranial lobe)
31 Primary fissure
32 Cerebellum (caudal lobe)
33 Transverse sinus
34 Occipital bone

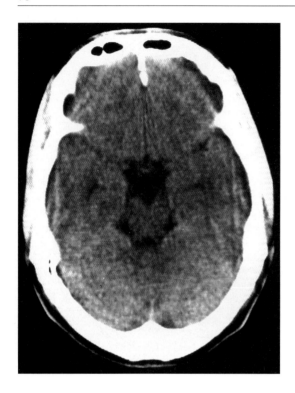

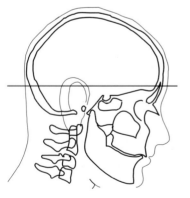

■ Frontal lobe
□ Temporal lobe
▥ Cerebellum
▤ Mesencephalon
▨ Pons

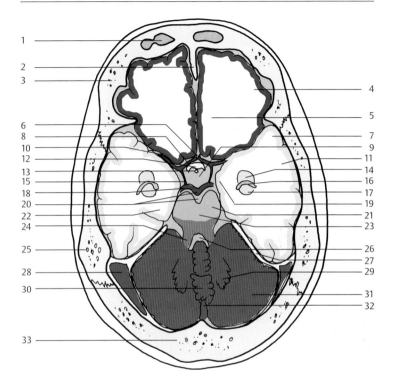

1   Frontal sinus
2   Falx cerebri
3   Frontal bone
4   Orbital gyri
5   Gyrus rectus
6   Anterior communicating artery
7   Superior temporal gyrus
8   Anterior cerebral artery
9   Pentagon of basal cisterns
10 Middle cerebral artery
11 Middle temporal gyrus
12 Optic chiasm
13 Infundibulum (pituitary stalk)
14 Amygdaloid body
15 Posterior communicating artery
16 Lateral ventricle (temporal horn)
17 Hippocampus
18 Posterior cerebral artery
19 Uncus
20 Basilar artery and interpeduncu-
    lar cistern
21 Cerebral peduncle
22 Parahippocampal gyrus
23 Pons
24 Cerebellar peduncle
25 Temporal bone
26 Fourth ventricle
27 Tentorium of cerebellum
28 Sigmoid sinus
29 Dentate nucleus
30 Vermis of cerebellum
31 Cerebellar hemisphere
32 Occipital sinus
33 Occipital bone

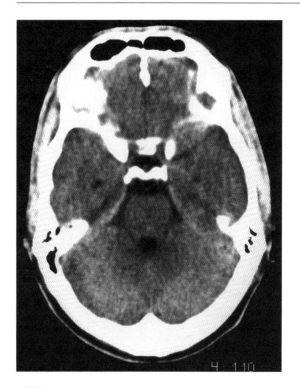

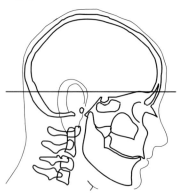

■ Frontal lobe
□ Temporal lobe
▨ Cerebellum
▨ Pons

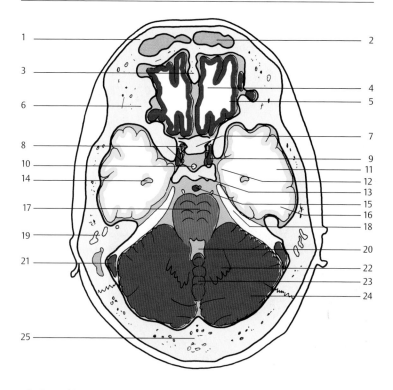

1 Frontal bone
2 Frontal sinus
3 Crista galli
4 Gyrus rectus
5 Orbital gyri
6 Sphenoid bone
7 Anterior clinoid process
8 Cavernous sinus
9 Internal carotid artery
10 Infundibulum (pituitary stalk)
11 Middle temporal gyrus
12 Parahippocampal gyrus
13 Posterior clinoid process
14 Lateral ventricle (temporal horn)
15 Basilar artery
16 Inferior temporal gyrus
17 Pons
18 Tentorium of cerebellum
19 Temporal bone
20 Fourth ventricle
21 Sigmoid sinus
22 Dentate nucleus
23 Vermis of cerebellum
24 Cerebellar hemisphere
25 Occipital bone

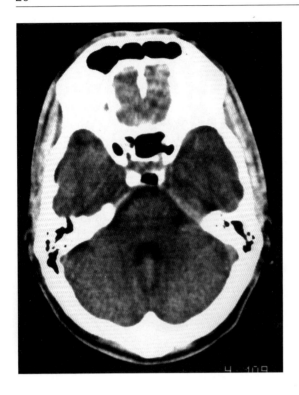

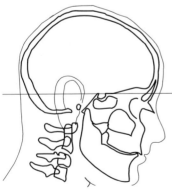

■ Frontal lobe
□ Temporal lobe
▥ Cerebellum
▨ Pons

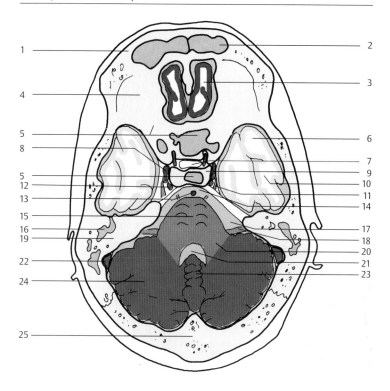

1   Frontal bone
2   Frontal sinus
3   Gyrus rectus
4   Sphenoid bone (lesser wing)
    and orbital roof
5   Sphenoid sinus
6   Temporal pole
7   Pituitary gland
8   Internal carotid artery
9   Dorsum sellae
10 Inferior temporal gyrus
11 Trigeminal nerve (ganglion)
12 Cavernous sinus
13 Basilar artery

14 Prepontine cistern
15 Pons
16 Mastoid antrum
17 Cerebellopontine angle cistern
18 Facial and vestibulocochlear
    nerves
19 Petrous part of temporal bone
20 Middle cerebellar peduncle
21 Fourth ventricle
22 Sigmoid sinus
23 Vermis of cerebellum
24 Cerebellum (caudal lobe)
25 Occipital bone

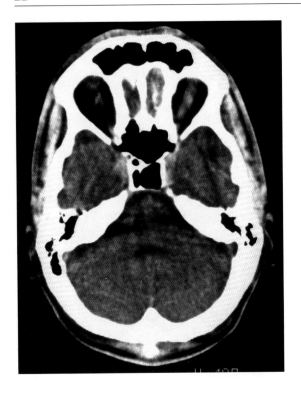

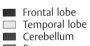

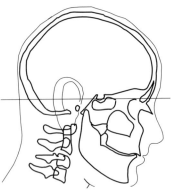

Frontal lobe
Temporal lobe
Cerebellum
Pons

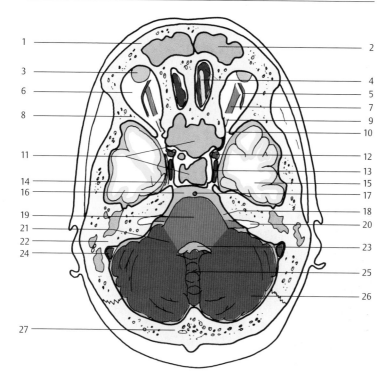

1 Frontal bone
2 Frontal sinus
3 Eyeball
4 Gyrus rectus, olfactory bulb
5 Ophthalmic vein
6 Orbit
7 Superior rectus muscle
8 Sphenoid bone
9 Optic nerve
10 Superior orbital fissure
11 Sphenoid sinus
12 Cavernous sinus
13 Internal carotid artery
14 Trigeminal nerve

15 Inferior temporal gyrus
16 Prepontine cistern
17 Basilar artery
18 Cerebellopontine angle cistern
19 Pons
20 Internal auditory canal
21 Middle and inferior cerebellar
   peduncles
22 Petrous part of temporal bone
23 Fourth ventricle
24 Sigmoid sinus
25 Vermis of cerebellum
26 Cerebellum (caudal lobe)
27 Occipital bone

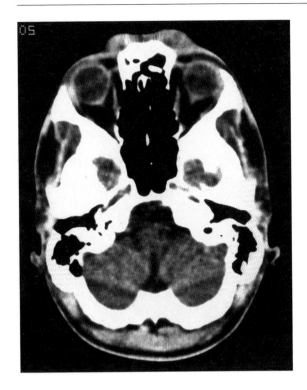

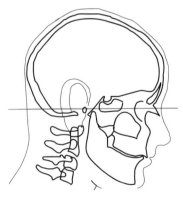

Temporal lobe
Cerebellum
Pons
Medulla oblongata

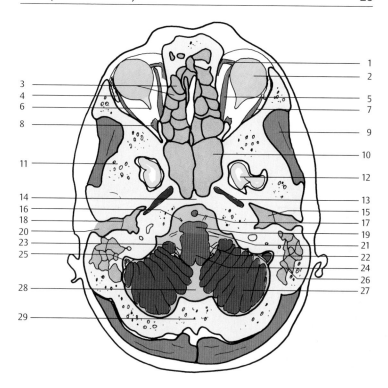

1 Superior oblique muscle
2 Eyeball
3 Ethmoid labyrinth
4 Lacrimal gland
5 Medial rectus muscle
6 Optic nerve
7 Lateral rectus muscle
8 Superior rectus muscle
9 Temporalis muscle
10 Sphenoid sinus
11 Temporal bone
12 Temporal lobe (base)
13 Internal carotid artery
14 Clivus
15 Tympanic cavity
16 Abducens nerve

17 Basilar artery
18 Tympanic membrane
19 Pons
20 External auditory canal
21 Anterior inferior cerebellar artery
22 Glossophanyngeal and vagus nerves
23 Floccule
24 Medulla oblongata
25 Sigmoid sinus
26 Mastoid air cells
27 Cerebellar hemisphere caudal lobe)
28 Cisterna magna (cerebello-medullary cistern)
29 Occipital bone

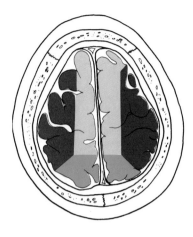
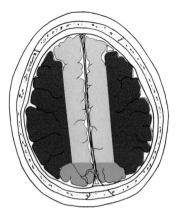
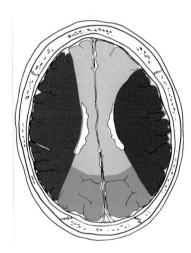
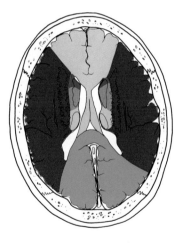

Anterior cerebral artery

☐ Terminal branches
■ Central branches

Middle cerebral artery

■ Terminal branches
▦ Central branches

Posterior cerebral artery

■ Terminal branches
☐ Central branches

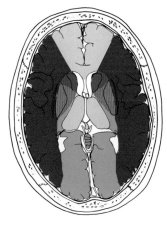
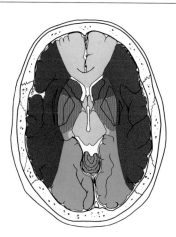
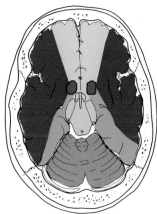
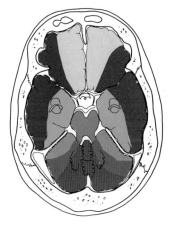

Anterior cerebral artery

Terminal branches
Central branches

Middle cerebral artery

Terminal branches
Central branches

Posterior cerebral artery

Terminal branches
Central branches

Superior cerebellar artery
Posterior inferior cerebellar artery
Anterior inferior cerebellar artery
Paramedian and circumferential arteries

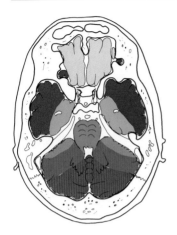

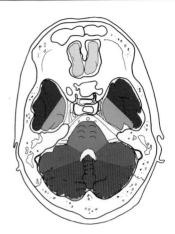

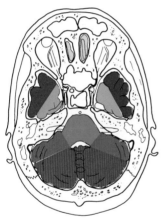

Anterior cerebral artery

- Terminal branches
- Central branches

Middle cerebral artery

- Terminal branches
- Central branches

Posterior cerebral artery

- Terminal branches
- Central branches

- Superior cerebellar artery
- Posterior inferior cerebellar artery
- Anterior inferior cerebellar artery
- Paramedian and circumferential arteries

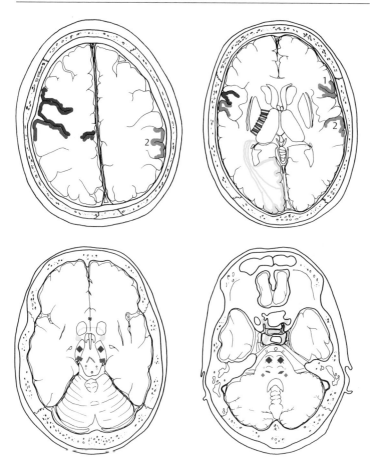

Motor system

Sensory system

Medial lemniscal tract
Spinothalamic tract
Mesencephalic nucleus of trigeminal nerve

Oculomotor nucleus and pathways
Optic tract
Speech center (1 = motor, 2 = sensory)

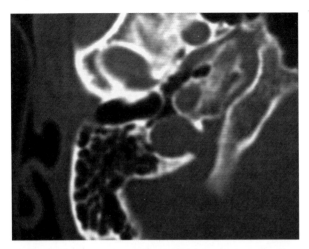

1

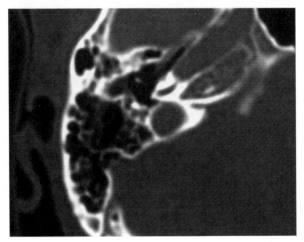

2

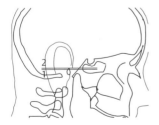

Frontal

Lateral ☐ Medial

Occipital

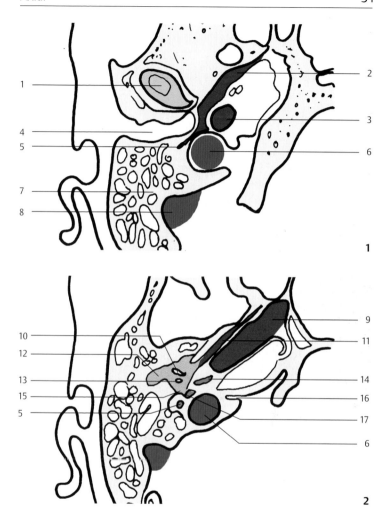

1

2

1 Temporomandibular joint
  (glenoid roof and articular disk)
2 Eustachian tube
3 Internal carotid artery
4 External auditory canal
5 Facial canal
6 Internal jugular vein
7 Mastoid process
8 Sigmoid sinus

9 Carotid canal
10 Malleus (manubrium)
11 Tensor tympani muscle (canal)
12 Middle ear
13 Incus (long crus)
14 Cochlea (basal turn)
15 Sinus tympani
16 Vestibular aqueduct
17 Round window

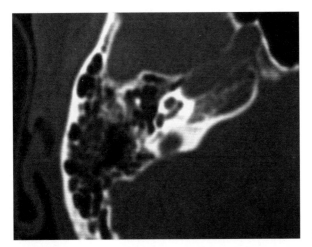

3

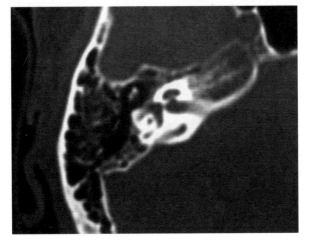

4

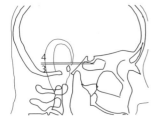

Frontal

Lateral ☐ Medial

Occipital

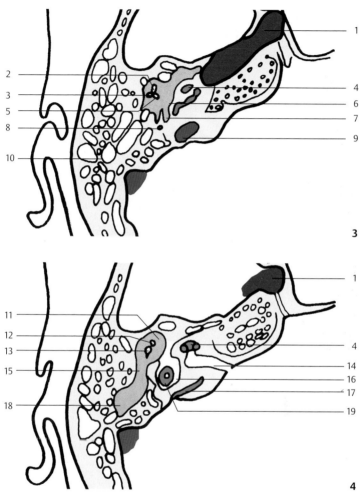

3

4

1 Internal carotid artery (canal)
2 Malleus (manubrium)
3 Incus (long crus)
4 Cochlea
5 Stapes
6 Oval window
7 Sinus tympani
8 Facial canal
9 Internal jugular vein (bulb)
10 Mastoid

11 Epitympanic recess
12 Malleus (head)
13 Incus (short crus)
14 Internal auditory canal
15 Aditus ad antrum
16 Vestibule
17 Posterior semicircular canal
18 Mastoid antrum
19 Lateral semicircular canal

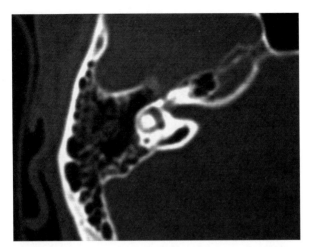

5

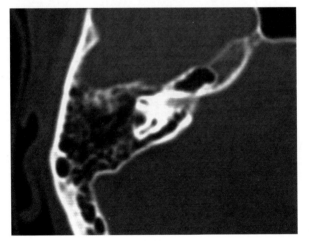

6

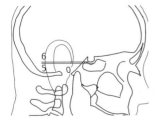

Frontal

Lateral ▢ Medial

Occipital

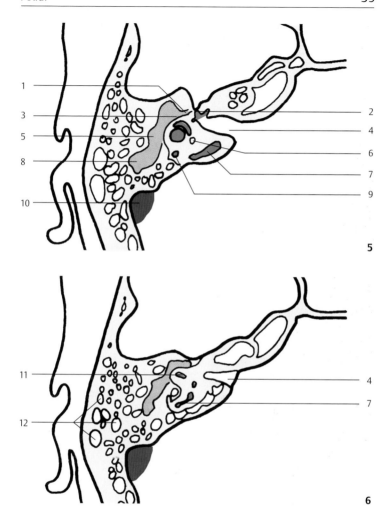

1 Geniculate ganglion
2 Facial nerve (first part)
3 Facial nerve (second part)
4 Internal auditory canal
5 Tympanic cavity
6 Vestibule
7 Posterior semicircular canal

8 Mastoid antrum
9 Lateral semicircular canal
10 Sigmoid sinus
11 Anterior (superior) semicircular canal
12 Mastoid air cells

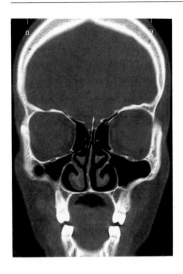

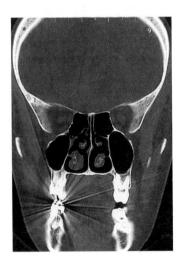

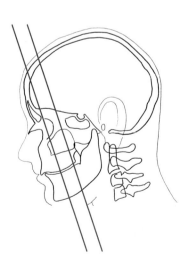

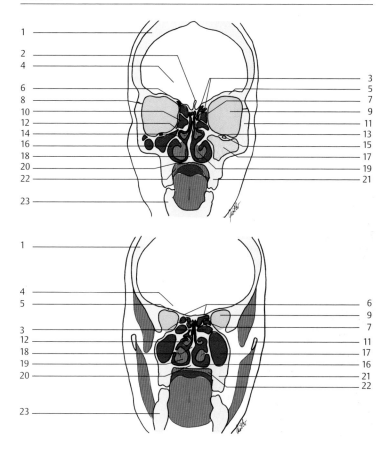

1	Frontal bone	**13**	Orbital floor
2	Crista galli	**14**	Middle nasal meatus
3	Ethmoid labyrinth	**15**	Infraorbital artery and vein
4	Anterior cranial fossa	**16**	Inferior nasal meatus
5	Orbital roof	**17**	Maxillary sinus
6	Cribriform plate	**18**	Nasal septum
7	Orbital plate of ethmoid bone	**19**	Inferior nasal turbinate
8	Frontozygomatic suture	**20**	Hard palate
9	Orbit	**21**	Maxilla
10	Ethmoid bulla	**22**	Soft palate
11	Zygomatic bone	**23**	Mandible
12	Middle nasal turbinate		

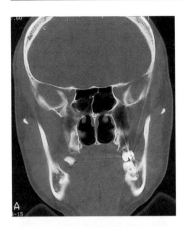

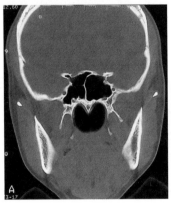

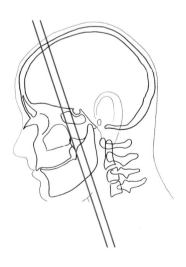

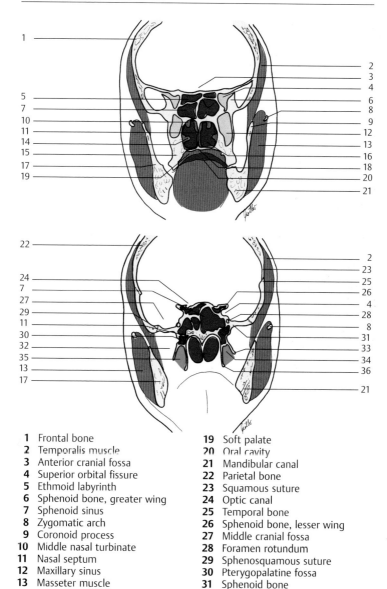

1   Frontal bone
2   Temporalis muscle
3   Anterior cranial fossa
4   Superior orbital fissure
5   Ethmoid labyrinth
6   Sphenoid bone, greater wing
7   Sphenoid sinus
8   Zygomatic arch
9   Coronoid process
10 Middle nasal turbinate
11 Nasal septum
12 Maxillary sinus
13 Masseter muscle
14 Inferior nasal turbinate
15 Maxilla
16 Inferior nasal meatus
17 Mandibular ramus
18 Hard palate

19 Soft palate
20 Oral cavity
21 Mandibular canal
22 Parietal bone
23 Squamous suture
24 Optic canal
25 Temporal bone
26 Sphenoid bone, lesser wing
27 Middle cranial fossa
28 Foramen rotundum
29 Sphenosquamous suture
30 Pterygopalatine fossa
31 Sphenoid bone
32 Lateral pterygoid muscle
33 Pterygoid process, lateral plate
34 Pterygoid fossa
35 Medial pterygoid muscle
36 Pterygoid process, medial plate

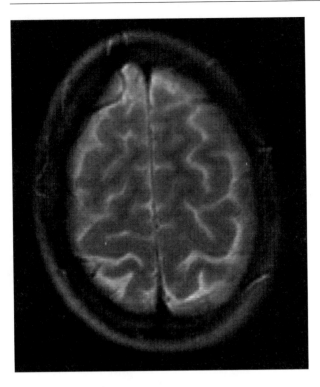

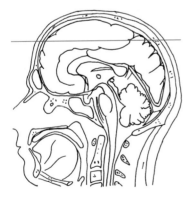

■ Frontal lobe
■ Parietal lobe

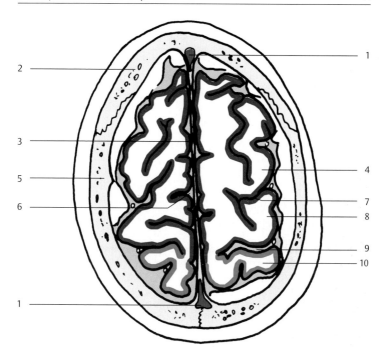

1 Superior sagittal sinus
2 Frontal bone
3 Falx cerebri
4 Middle frontal gyrus
5 Parietal bone

6 Superior longitudinal fissure
7 Precentral sulcus
8 Precentral gyrus
9 Central sulcus
10 Postcentral gyrus

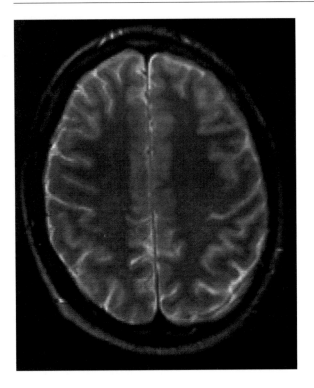

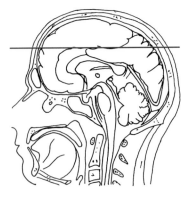

■ Frontal lobe
■ Parietal lobe

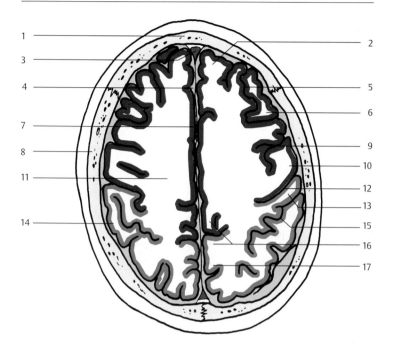

1   Frontal bone
2   Superior frontal gyrus
3   Superior sagittal sinus
4   Longitudinal fissure
5   Superior frontal sulcus
6   Middle frontal gyrus
7   Falx cerebri
8   Parietal bone
9   Precentral sulcus

10   Precentral gyrus
11   Cerebral white matter
12   Central sulcus
13   Postcentral gyrus
14   Parietal lobule
15   Postcentral sulcus
16   Paracentral lobule
17   Precuneus

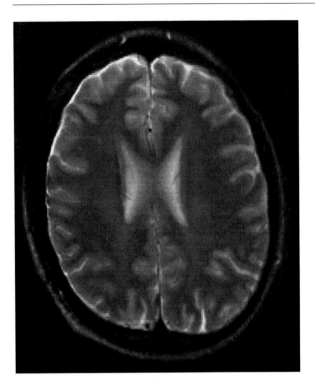

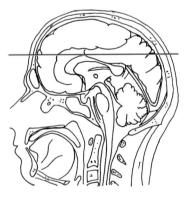

■ Frontal lobe
■ Parietal lobe
■ Occipital lobe

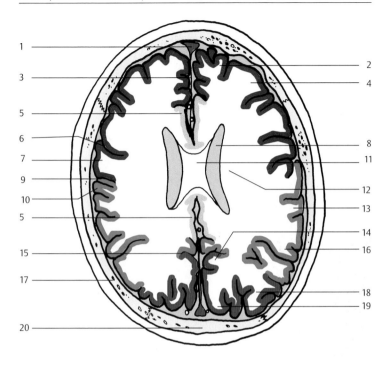

1 Superior sagittal sinus
2 Superior frontal gyrus
3 Falx cerebri
4 Middle frontal gyrus
5 Cingulum
6 Precentral sulcus
7 Precentral gyrus
8 Lateral ventricle (central part)
9 Central sulcus
10 Postcentral gyrus

11 Corpus callosum
12 Corona radiata
13 Supramarginal gyrus
14 Precuneus
15 Parietooccipital sulcus
16 Angular gyrus
17 Parietal bone
18 Occipital gyri
19 Cuneus
20 Occipital bone

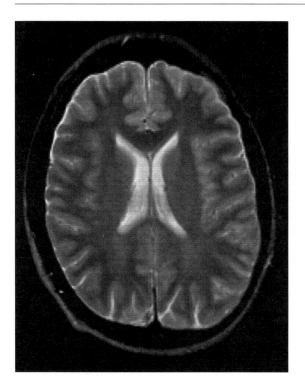

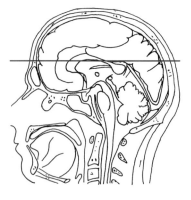

■ Frontal lobe
☐ Temporal lobe
▨ Parietal lobe
▦ Occipital lobe

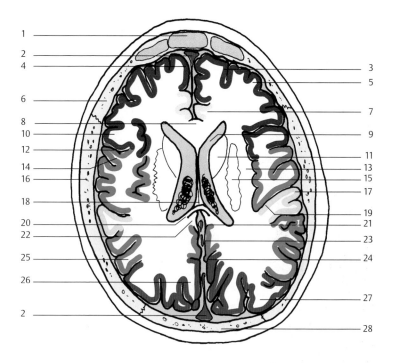

1 Frontal sinus
2 Superior sagittal sinus
3 Superior frontal gyrus
4 Falx cerebri
5 Middle frontal gyrus
6 Frontal bone
7 Cingulate gyrus
8 Corpus callosum
9 Lateral ventricle (anterior horn)
10 Precentral gyrus
11 Caudate nucleus (head)
12 Central sulcus
13 Insula
14 Postcentral gyrus

15 Corona radiata
16 Parietal bone
17 Superior temporal gyrus
18 Fornix (body)
19 Lateral sulcus
20 Corpus callosum (splenium)
21 Great cerebral vein
22 Cingulate gyrus
23 Straight sinus
24 Parietooccipital sulcus
25 Angular gyrus
26 Cuneus
27 Occipital gyri
28 Occipital bone

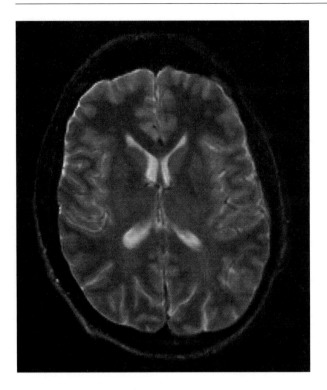

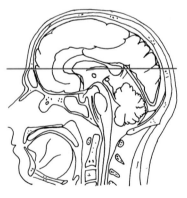

■ Frontal lobe
□ Temporal lobe
■ Parietal lobe
■ Occipital lobe

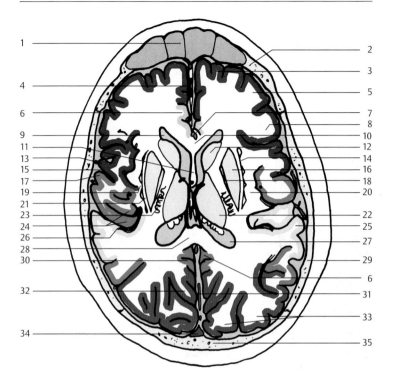

1 Frontal sinus
2 Frontal bone
3 Superior frontal gyrus
4 Falx cerebri and interhemispheric fissure
5 Middle frontal gyrus
6 Cingulate gyrus
7 Pericallosal artery
8 Inferior frontal gyrus
9 Lateral ventricle (anterior horn)
10 Corpus callosum (genu)
11 Septum pellucidum
12 Caudate nucleus (head)
13 Precentral gyrus
14 Claustrum
15 Central sulcus
16 Putamen
17 Postcentral gyrus
18 Globus pallidus
19 Capsula extrema
20 Insula
21 External capsule
22 Thalamus
23 Internal capsule
24 Transverse temporal gyrus
25 Superior temporal gyrus
26 Lateral sulcus
27 Lateral ventricle (trigone)
28 Corpus callosum (splenium)
29 Parietal bone
30 Parietooccipital sulcus
31 Straight sinus
32 Cuneus
33 Occipital gyri
34 Superior sagittal sinus
35 Occipital bone

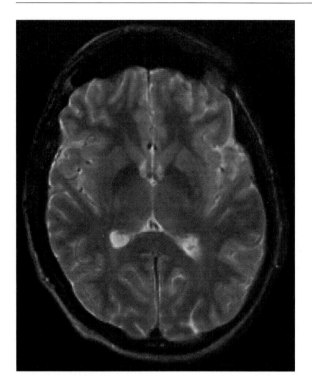

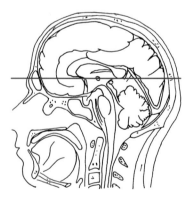

■ Frontal lobe
☐ Temporal lobe
▓ Parietal lobe
■ Occipital lobe

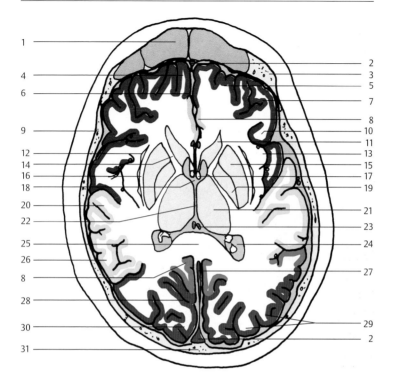

1 Frontal sinus
2 Superior sagittal sinus
3 Frontal bone
4 Frontal pole
5 Superior frontal gyrus
6 Falx cerebri and interhemispheric fissure
7 Middle frontal gyrus
8 Cingulate gyrus
9 Parietal bone
10 Frontal operculum
11 Caudate nucleus (head)
12 Claustrum
13 Insula
14 Internal capsule (anterior limb)
15 Putamen
16 External capsule

17 Fornix (anterior column)
18 Interventricular foramen (of Monro)
19 Globus pallidus
20 Superior temporal gyrus
21 Thalamus
22 Third ventricle
23 Posterior choroidal artery
24 Lateral ventricle (trigone)
25 Corpus callosum (splenium)
26 Middle temporal gyrus
27 Straight sinus
28 Calcarine sulcus
29 Occipital gyri
30 Occipital pole
31 Occipital bone

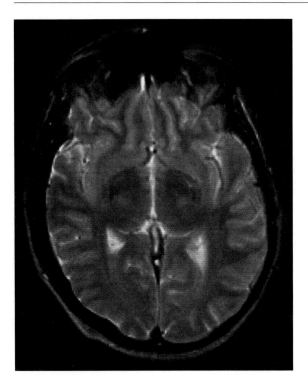

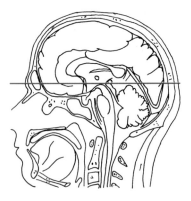

Frontal lobe
Temporal lobe
Occipital lobe

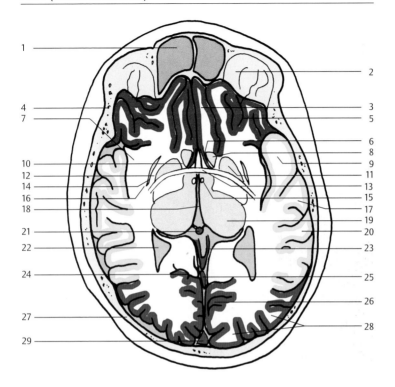

1 Frontal sinus
2 Orbital roof
3 Gyrus rectus
4 Frontal bone
5 Orbital gyri
6 Anterior cerebral artery
7 Insula
8 Caudate nucleus (head)
9 Superior temporal gyrus
10 Internal capsule
11 Putamen
12 External capsule
13 Anterior commissure
14 Claustrum
15 Fornix (postcommissural)
16 Capsula extrema
17 Middle temporal gyrus
18 Third ventricle
19 Thalamus
20 Inferior temporal gyrus
21 Pineal gland
22 Lateral ventricle (trigone)
23 Internal cerebral vein
24 Parietooccipital sulcus
25 Great cerebral vein
26 Striate cortex
27 Occipital bone
28 Occipital gyri
29 Superior sagittal sinus

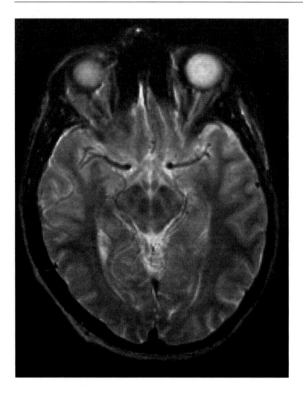

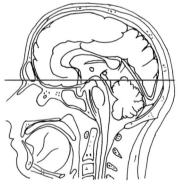

■ Frontal lobe
□ Temporal lobe
■ Occipital lobe
■ Cerebellum
□ Mesencephalon

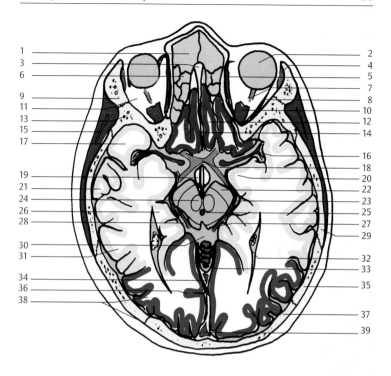

1 Frontal sinus
2 Eyeball
3 Crista galli
4 Lacrimal gland
5 Superior oblique muscle
6 Ethmoid labyrinth
7 Optic nerve
8 Lateral rectus muscle
9 Zygomatic bone
10 Superior rectus muscle
11 Orbit
12 Gyrus rectus
13 Sphenoid bone
14 Anterior cerebral artery
15 Temporalis muscle
16 Middle cerebral artery
17 Superior temporal gyrus
18 Optic chiasm
19 Hypothalamus
20 Cuneus

21 Middle temporal gyrus
22 Cerebral peduncle
23 Posterior cerebral artery
24 Red nucleus
25 Aqueduct
26 Hippocampus
27 Cranial colliculus
28 Ambient cistern
29 Temporal bone
30 Cistern of great cerebral vein
31 Inferior temporal gyrus
32 Lateral ventricle (temporal horn)
33 Cranial lobe of cerebellum
34 Straight sinus
35 Parietal bone
36 Calcarine sulcus
37 Occipital bone
38 Occipital gyri
39 Superior sagittal sinus

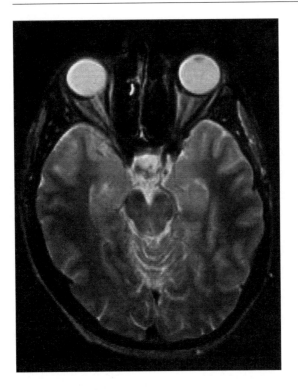

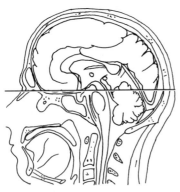

■ Frontal lobe
☐ Temporal lobe
▨ Cerebellum
▨ Mesencephalon

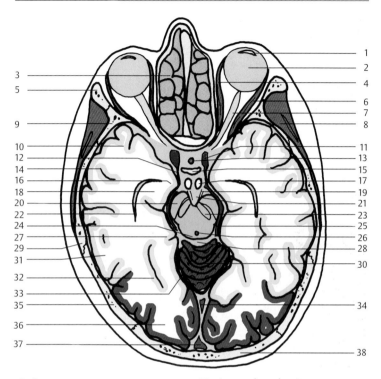

1 Lens
2 Eyeball
3 Ethmoid labyrinth
4 Medial rectus muscle
5 Zygomatic bone
6 Lateral rectus muscle
7 Optic nerve
8 Temporalis muscle
9 Sphenoid bone
10 Superior temporal gyrus
11 Internal carotid artery
12 Posterior communicating artery
13 Pituitary stalk
14 Middle temporal gyrus
15 Dorsum sellae
16 Uncus
17 Mamillary body
18 Hippocampus
19 Oculomotor nerve
20 Cerebral peduncle

21 Interpeduncular cistern
22 Lateral ventricle (temporal horn)
23 Substantia nigra
24 Caudal colliculus
25 Posterior cerebral artery
   (in ambient cistern)
26 Aqueduct
27 Parahippocampal gyrus
28 Quadrigeminal cistern
29 Temporal bone
30 Cranial lobe of cerebellum
31 Inferior temporal gyrus
32 Collateral sulcus
33 Tentorium
34 Straight sinus
35 Parietal bone
36 Occipital gyri
37 Superior sagittal sinus
38 Occipital bone

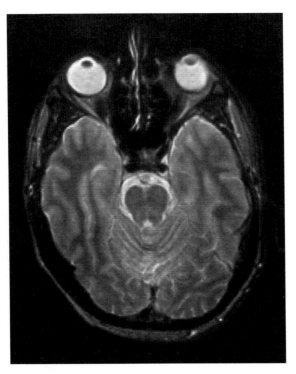

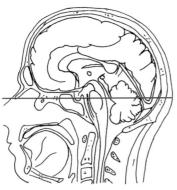

☐ Temporal lobe
■ Occipital lobe
■ Cerebellum
▨ Mesencephalon
▨ Pons

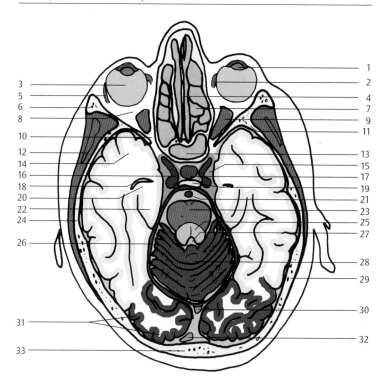

1 Lens
2 Medial rectus muscle
3 Eyeball
4 Nasal septum
5 Lateral rectus muscle
6 Zygomatic bone
7 Ethmoid labyrinth
8 Orbit
9 Inferior rectus muscle
10 Superior orbital fissure
11 Sphenoid bone
12 Temporalis muscle
13 Sphenoid sinus
14 Temporal lobe
15 Cavernous sinus
16 Internal carotid artery
17 Pituitary
18 Lateral ventricle (temporal horn)
19 Dorsum sellae
20 Hippocampus
21 Basilar artery
22 Parahippocampal gyrus
23 Pons
24 Temporal bone
25 Reticular formation
26 Tentorium of cerebellum
27 Fourth ventricle
28 Cranial lobe of cerebellum
29 Parietal bone
30 Straight sinus
31 Occipital gyri
32 Superior sagittal sinus
33 Occipital bone

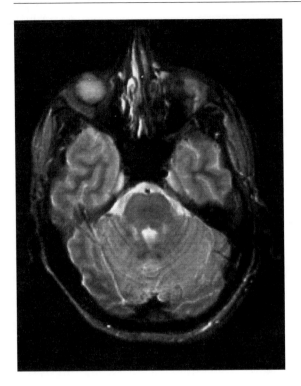

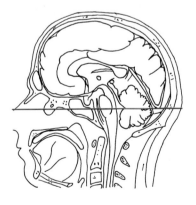

Temporal lobe
Occipital lobe
Cerebellum
Pons

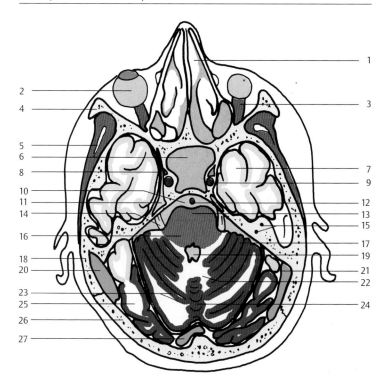

1 Nasal cavity
2 Eyeball
3 Inferior rectus muscle
4 Zygomatic bone
5 Temporalis muscle
6 Sphenoid sinus
7 Temporal lobe
8 Cavernous sinus
9 Internal carotid artery
10 Cerebellopontine angle cistern
11 Trigeminal (gasserian) ganglion in trigeminal cavity (Meckel's cave)
12 Basilar artery
13 Pons

14 Trigeminal nerve (cranial nerve V)
15 Anterior semicircular canal
16 Middle cerebellar peduncle
17 Cerebellum (cranial lobe)
18 Temporal bone
19 Fourth ventricle
20 Transverse sinus
21 Tentorium of cerebellum
22 Dentate nucleus
23 Cerebellum (caudal lobe)
24 Nodule of vermis
25 Occipital pole
26 Occipital bone
27 Sinus confluence

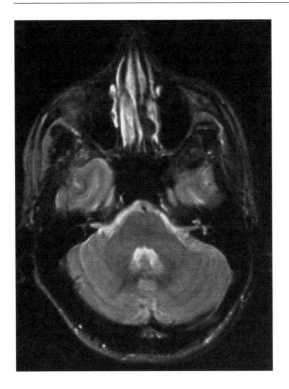

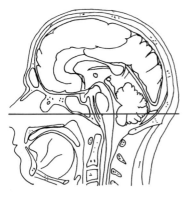

☐ Temporal lobe
▓ Cerebellum
▓ Pons

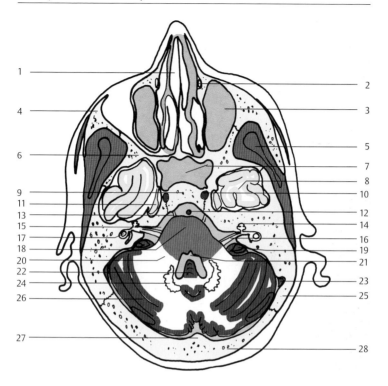

1 Nasal septum
2 Nasolacrimal duct
3 Maxillary sinus
4 Zygomatic bone
5 Temporalis muscle
6 Sphenoid bone
7 Sphenoid sinus
8 Temporal lobe (base)
9 Clivus
10 Internal carotid artery
11 Trigeminal (gasserian) ganglion
12 Basilar artery
13 Abducens nerve (cranial nerve VI)
14 Cochlea
15 Cerebellopontine angle cistern

16 Vestibulocochlear nerve (cranial nerve VIII)
17 Semicircular canal
18 Pons
19 Floccule
20 Middle cerebellar peduncle
21 Fourth ventricle
22 Nodule of vermis
23 Sigmoid sinus
24 Dentate nucleus
25 Temporal bone
26 Cerebellum (caudal lobe)
27 Internal occipital protuberance
28 Occipital bone

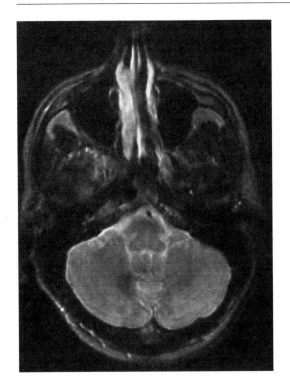

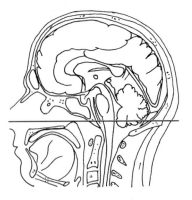

■ Cerebellum
■ Pons
■ Medulla oblongata

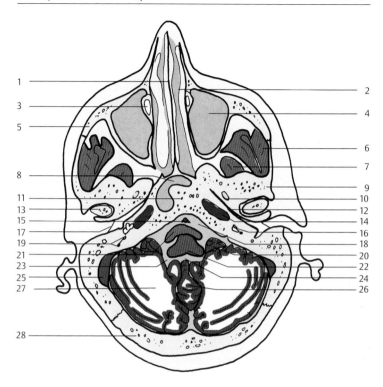

1 Nasal septum	**15** Basilar artery
2 Nasal cavity	**16** Cochlea
3 Nasolacrimal duct	**17** External auditory canal
4 Maxillary sinus	**18** Prepontine cistern
5 Zygomatic bone	**19** Posterior semicircular canal
6 Temporalis muscle	**20** Floccule
7 Lateral pterygoid muscle	**21** Pons
8 Sphenoid sinus	**22** Medulla oblongata
9 Temporal bone	**23** Foramina of Luschka
10 Mandibular nerve (third division of trigeminal)	**24** Fourth ventricle
11 Clivus	**25** Sigmoid sinus
12 Eustachian tube	**26** Uvula of cerebellum
13 Temporomandibular joint	**27** Caudal lobe of cerebellum
14 Internal carotid artery	**28** Occipital bone

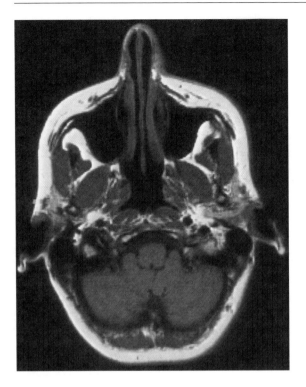

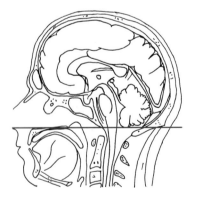

Cerebellum
Medulla oblongata

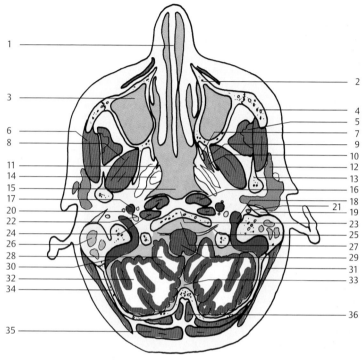

1 Nasal septum
2 Maxilla
3 Maxillary sinus
4 Zygomatic bone
5 Temporalis muscle
6 Masseter muscle
7 Medial pterygoid process
8 Lateral pterygoid muscle
9 Lateral pterygoid process
10 Medial pterygoid and tensor veli palatini muscles
11 Pharyngeal orifice of eustachian tube
12 Parotid gland
13 Mandibular condyle
14 Eustachian tube
15 Nasopharynx
16 Longus capitis muscle
17 Internal carotid artery
18 Internal jugular vein (bulb)
19 Styloid process

20 Glossopharyngeal nerve (cranial nerve IX)
21 Facial nerve (cranial nerve VII)
22 Vagus nerve (cranial nerve X)
23 Clivus
24 Rectus capitis anterior muscle
25 Hypoglossal nerve (cranial nerve XII)
26 Mastoid process
27 Premedullary cistern
28 Cerebellar tonsil
29 Medulla oblongata (with central canal)
30 Sigmoid sinus
31 Splenius capitis muscle
32 Cerebellum (posterior caudal lobe)
33 Cisterna magna
34 Occipital bone
35 Semispinalis capitis muscle
36 Rectus capitis posterior muscles (minor and major)

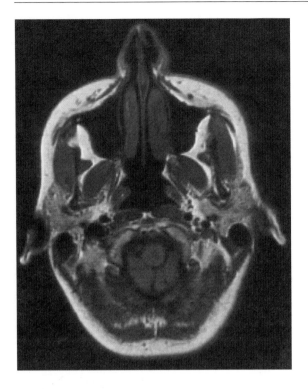

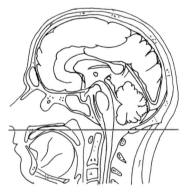

■ Cerebellum
▥ Medulla oblongata

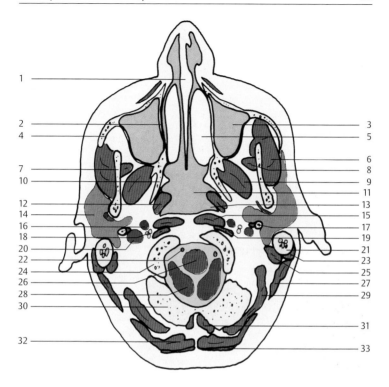

1 Nasal septum
2 Medial wall of maxillary sinus
3 Maxillary sinus
4 Zygomatic bone (arch)
5 Nasal turbinate
6 Masseter muscle
7 Mandible
8 Temporalis muscle
9 Lateral pterygoid muscle
10 Pterygoid process
11 Nasopharynx
12 Eustachian tube
13 Lateral pharyngeal recess
    (Rosenmüller's fossa)
14 Parotid gland
15 Longus capitis muscle
16 Internal carotid artery
17 Styloid process and styloid muscles
18 Cranial nerves X, XI and XII
    (vagus, accessory, hypoglossal)
19 Rectus capitis anterior muscle
20 Internal jugular vein
21 Mastoid process
22 Vertebral artery
23 Sternocleidomastoid muscle
24 Occipital condyle
25 Digastric muscle (posterior belly)
26 Medulla oblongata
27 Splenius capitis muscle
28 Cerebellar tonsil
29 Rectus capitis posterior muscle
    (major)
30 Occipital bone
31 Rectus capitis posterior muscle
    (minor)
32 Semispinalis capitis muscle
33 Trapezius muscle

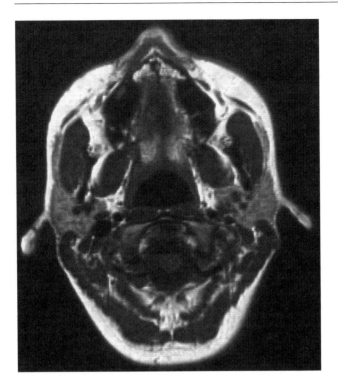

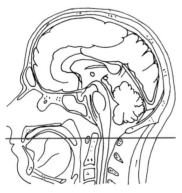

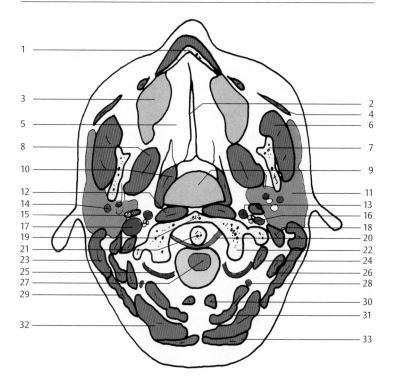

1 Incisive bone

2 Nasal crest

3 Maxillary sinus

4 Zygomatic muscle

5 Palatine bone and process

6 Masseter muscle

7 Mandible (ramus)

8 Medial pterygoid muscle

9 Nasopharynx

10 Levator veli palatini muscle

11 Parotid gland

12 Longus capitis muscle

13 Internal carotid artery

14 Retromandibular vein

15 Styloid process

16 Cranial nerves X, XI, and XII (vagus, accessory, hypoglossal)

17 Internal jugular vein

18 Digastric muscle (posterior belly)

19 Atlas (anterior arch)

20 Cruciform ligament of atlas

21 Dens of axis

22 Atlas (lateral mass)

23 Sternocleidomastoid muscle

24 Inferior oblique muscle

25 Vertebral artery

26 Longissimus capitis muscle

27 Spinal cord

28 Deep cervical vein

29 Splenius capitis muscle

30 Rectus capitis posterior muscle (minor)

31 Rectus capitis posterior muscle (major)

32 Semispinalis capitis muscle

33 Trapezius muscle

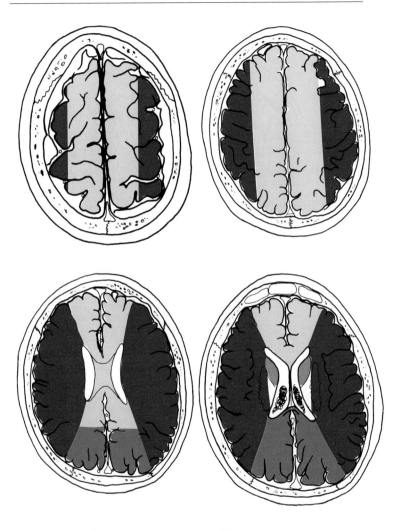

Anterior cerebral artery
- Terminal branches
- Central branches

Middle cerebral artery
- Terminal branches
- Central branches

Posterior cerebral artery
- Terminal branches
- Central branches

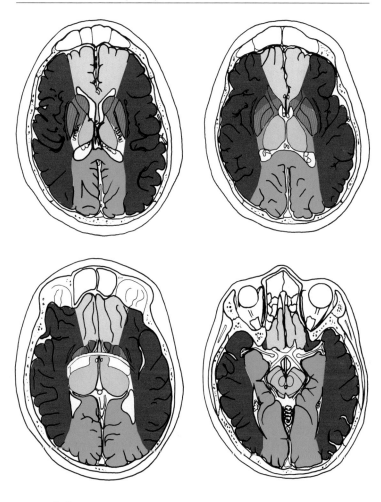

Cerebellum

■ Superior cerebellar artery
▨ Posterior inferior cerebellar artery
■ Anterior inferior cerebellar artery
■ Paramedian and circumferential arteries

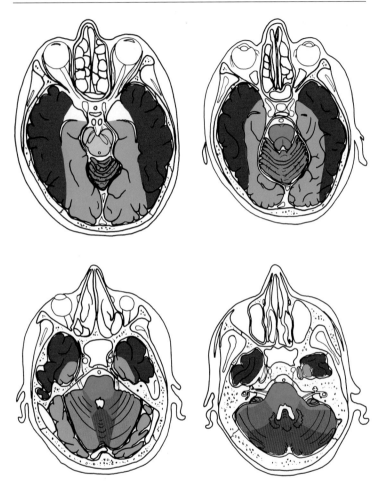

Anterior cerebral artery
☐ Terminal branches
▨ Central branches

Middle cerebral artery
▨ Terminal branches
▨ Central branches

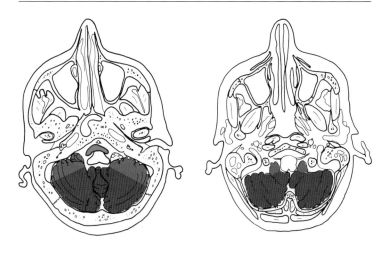

Posterior cerebral artery

- Terminal branches
- Central branches

Cerebellum

- Superior cerebellar artery
- Posterior inferior cerebellar artery
- Anterior inferior cerebellar artery
- Paramedian and circumferential arteries

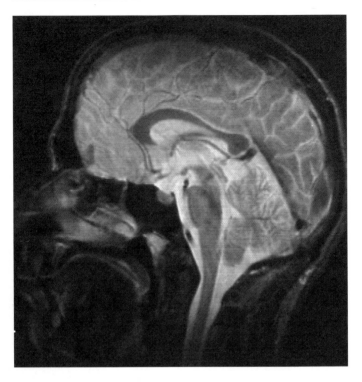

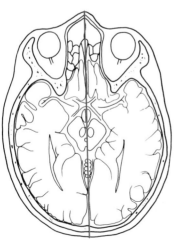

■ Frontal lobe
▨ Parietal lobe
■ Occipital lobe
▥ Cerebellum
▨ Mesencephalon
▥ Pons
▥ Medulla oblongata

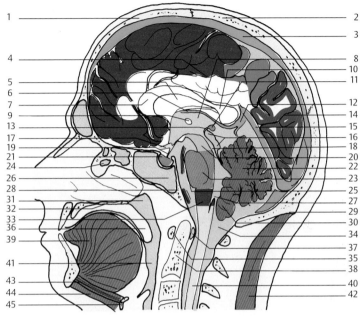

1 Frontal bone
2 Parietal bone
3 Superior sagittal sinus
4 Cingulate sulcus
5 Septum pellucidum
6 Internal cerebral vein
7 Corpus callosum (genu)
8 Third ventricle
9 Interthalamic adhesion
10 Corpus callosum (splenium)
11 Pineal gland
12 Great cerebral vein
13 Anterior and posterior commissures
14 Parietooccipital sulcus
15 Straight sinus
16 Cranial and caudal colliculi
17 Optic nerve
18 Aqueduct
19 Pituitary stalk
20 Tegmentum of mesencephalon
21 Pituitary gland
22 Cerebellum
23 Pons
24 Ethmoid labyrinth

25 Basilar artery
26 Sphenoid sinus
27 Fourth ventricle
28 Clivus
29 Occipital bone (external occipital protuberance)
30 Uvula of cerebellum
31 Nasopharynx
32 Hard palate
33 Medulla oblongata
34 Cisterna magna (cerebellomedullary cistern)
35 Atlas (arch)
36 Uvula
37 Transverse ligament of atlas
38 Dens of axis
39 Genioglossus muscle
40 Spinal cord
41 Oropharynx
42 Semispinalis capitis muscle
43 Geniohyoid muscle
44 Mylohyoid muscle
45 Hyoid bone

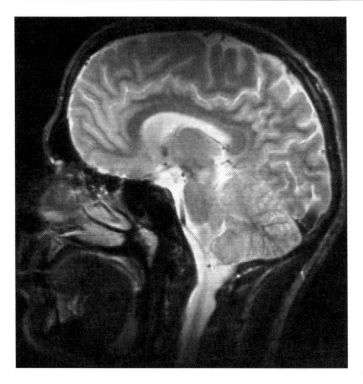

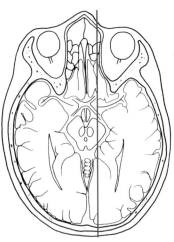

- Frontal lobe
- Parietal lobe
- Occipital lobe
- Cerebellum
- Mesencephalon
- Pons
- Medulla oblongata

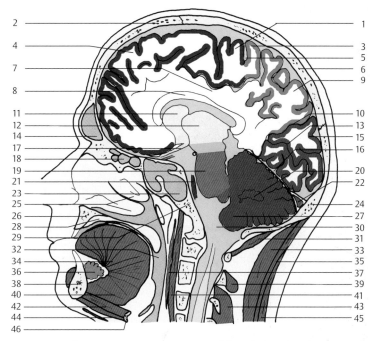

1 Precentral gyrus
2 Frontal bone
3 Postcentral gyrus
4 Superior frontal gyrus
5 Central sulcus
6 Parietal bone
7 Cingulum
8 Corpus callosum (trunk)
9 Precuneus
10 Parietooccipital sulcus
11 Caudate nucleus
12 Thalamus
13 Calcarine sulcus
14 Frontal sinus
15 Occipital gyri
16 Tentorium of cerebellum
17 Optic nerve
18 Ethmoid labyrinth
19 Pons
20 Dentate nucleus
21 Basilar artery
22 Transverse sinus
23 Sphenoid sinus
24 Occipital bone

25 Middle and inferior nasal turbinates
26 Maxilla
27 Cerebellar tonsil
28 Hard palate
29 Clivus
30 Cisterna magna
     (cerebellomedullary cistern)
31 Rectus capitis posterior muscle
     (minor)
32 Oropharynx
33 Semispinalis capitis muscle
34 Genioglossus muscle
35 Splenius capitis muscle
36 Sublingual gland
37 Pharyngeal constrictor muscle
38 Mandible (body)
39 Rectus capitis posterior muscle
40 Hyoglossus muscle
41 Longus capitis muscle
42 Geniohyoid muscle
43 Semispinalis cervicis muscle
44 Mylohyoid muscle
45 Trapezius muscle
46 Hyoid bone

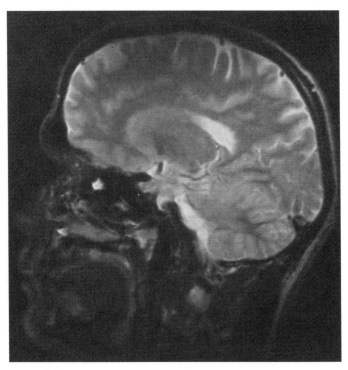

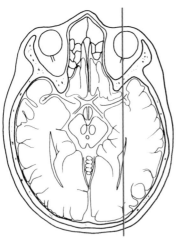

■ Frontal lobe
☐ Temporal lobe
■ Parietal lobe
■ Occipital lobe
■ Cerebellum
▨ Pons

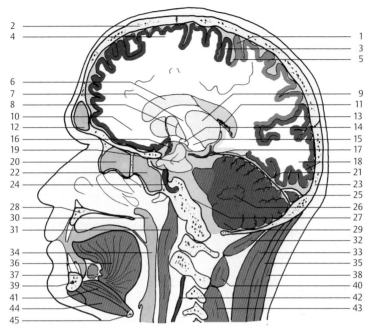

1 Postcentral gyrus
2 Frontal bone
3 Precentral gyrus
4 Superior frontal gyrus
5 Central sulcus
6 Caudate nucleus
7 Internal capsule
8 Lentiform nucleus
9 Thalamus
10 Orbital gyri
11 Lateral ventricle (choroid plexus)
12 Frontal sinus
13 Parietooccipital sulcus
14 Optic tract
15 Cerebral peduncle
16 Middle cerebral artery
17 Posterior cerebral artery
18 Occipital gyri
19 Uncus of hippocampal gyrus
20 Ethmoid labyrinth (posterior cells)
21 Tentorium of cerebellum
22 Sphenoid sinus
23 Occipital bone

24 Internal carotid artery
25 Transverse sinus
26 Dentate nucleus
27 Clivus
28 Hard palate
29 Cerebellar tonsil
30 Nasopharynx
31 Longus capitis muscle
32 Rectus capitis posterior muscle (major)
33 Semispinalis capitis muscle
34 Oropharynx
35 Splenius capitis muscle
36 Genioglossus muscle
37 Sublingual gland
38 Trapezius muscle
39 Mandible (body)
40 Obliquus capitis inferior muscle
41 Geniohyoid muscle
42 Vertebral artery
43 Semispinalis cervicis muscle
44 Mylohyoid muscle
45 Hyoid bone

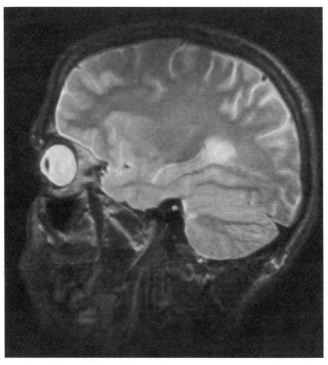

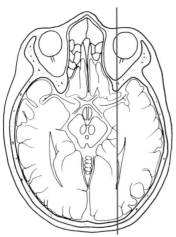

- Frontal lobe
- Temporal lobe
- Parietal lobe
- Occipital lobe
- Cerebellum

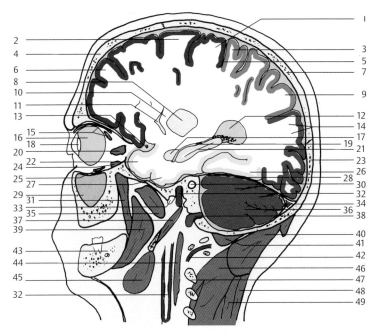

1	Precentral gyrus	25	Inferior rectus muscle
2	Superior frontal gyrus	26	Medial occipitotemporal gyrus
3	Postcentral gyrus	27	Inferior temporal gyrus
4	Frontal bone	28	Tentorium of cerebellum
5	Central sulcus	29	Maxillary sinus
6	Frontal gyri	30	Internal auditory canal
7	Parietal bone	31	Temporalis muscle
8	Globus pallidus	32	Internal carotid artery
9	Angular gyrus	33	Eustachian tube
10	Internal capsule	34	Transverse sinus
11	Putamen	35	Lateral pterygoid muscle
12	Lateral ventricle	36	Cerebellum (hemisphere)
13	Middle cerebral artery	37	Stylohyoid muscle
14	Occipital gyri	38	Internal jugular vein
15	Superior rectus and levator palpebrae superioris muscles	39	Medial pterygoid muscle
16	Eyeball	40	Splenius capitis muscle
17	Amygdaloid body	41	Rectus capitis muscle
18	Lens	42	Vertebral artery
19	Lateral ventricle (temporal horn)	43	Mandible
20	Lateral rectus muscle	44	Longus colli muscle
21	Hippocampus	45	Digastric muscle (posterior belly)
22	Middle temporal gyrus	46	Multifidus muscles
23	Occipital bone	47	Transverse processes
24	Orbital muscle	48	Trapezius muscle
		49	Levator scapulae muscle

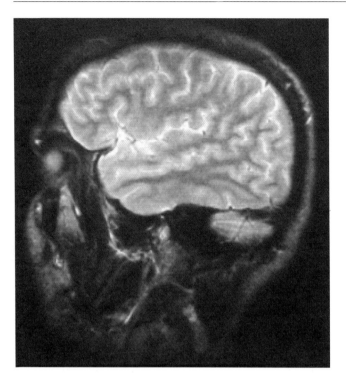

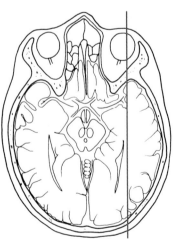

■ Frontal lobe
☐ Temporal lobe
▨ Parietal lobe
▨ Occipital lobe
■ Cerebellum

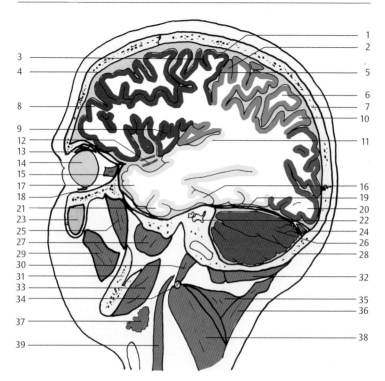

1 Precentral gyrus
2 Postcentral gyrus
3 Precentral sulcus
4 Frontal bone
5 Central sulcus
6 Supramarginal gyrus
7 Parietal bone
8 Inferior frontal gyrus
9 Insular cortex
10 Angular gyrus
11 Transverse temporal gyri
   (Heschl's gyrus)
12 Lateral sulcus and insular arteries
13 Levator palpebrae superioris muscle
14 Eyeball
15 Lateral rectus muscle
16 Lateral occipitotemporal gyrus
17 Middle temporal gyrus
18 Inferior oblique muscle
19 Tentorium of cerebellum

20 Occipital gyri
21 Inferior temporal gyrus
22 Cochlea
23 Maxillary sinus
24 Transverse sinus
25 Temporalis muscle
26 Cerebellum (caudal lobe)
27 Lateral pterygoid muscle
28 Occipital bone
29 Masseter muscle
30 Rectus capitis lateralis muscle
31 Mandible
32 Obliquus capitis muscle
33 Medial pterygoid muscle
34 Atlas (transverse process)
35 Longissimus capitis muscle
36 Splenius capitis muscle
37 Submandibular gland
38 Levator scapulae muscle
39 Jugular vein

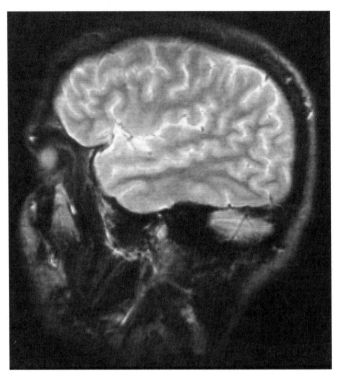

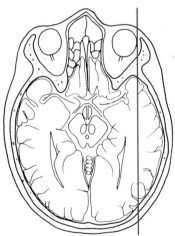

■ Frontal lobe
☐ Temporal lobe
▨ Parietal lobe
▨ Cerebellum

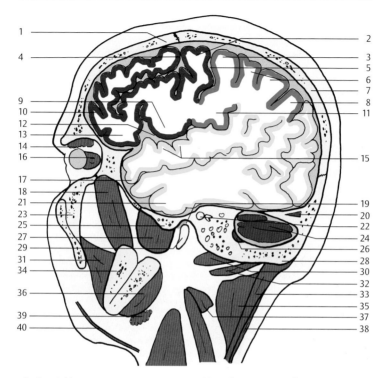

1 Frontal bone
2 Precentral gyrus
3 Postcentral gyrus
4 Precentral sulcus
5 Central sulcus
6 Supramarginal gyrus
7 Parietal bone
8 Angular gyrus
9 Frontal operculum
10 Inferior frontal gyrus
11 Parietal operculum
12 Lateral sulcus
13 Orbital gyri
14 Lacrimal gland
15 Temporal operculum
16 Lateral rectus muscle
17 Middle temporal gyrus
18 Temporalis muscle
19 Articular disk in glenoid fossa
20 Transverse sinus

21 Inferior temporal gyrus
22 Cochlea
23 Zygomatic bone
24 Cerebellum (caudal lobe)
25 Articular tubercle
26 Sigmoid sinus
27 Lateral pterygoid muscle
28 Occipital bone
29 Mandibular condyle
30 Rectus capitis lateralis muscle
31 Masseter muscle
32 Digastric muscle
33 Splenius capitis muscle
34 Mandible
35 Longissimus capitis muscle
36 Medial pterygoid muscle
37 Levator scapulae muscle
38 Trapezius muscle
39 Submandibular gland
40 Platysma

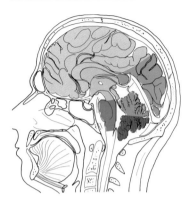
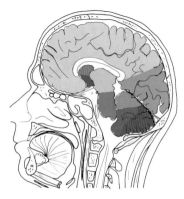
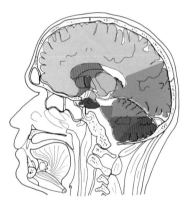
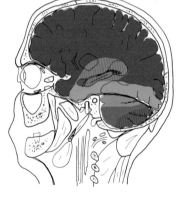

Anterior cerebral artery

▢ Terminal branches
■ Central branches

Middle cerebral artery

■ Terminal branches
▨ Central branches

Posterior cerebral artery

▢ Terminal branches
▢ Central branches

▨ Superior cerebellar artery
▨ Anterior inferior cerebellar artery
■ Posterior inferior cerebellar artery
■ Paramedian and circumferential arteries

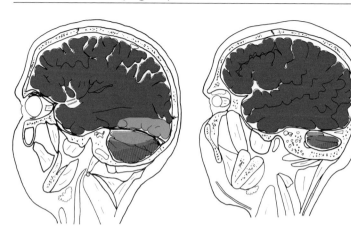

Middle cerebral artery
- Terminal branches

Posterior cerebral artery
- Terminal branches

- Superior cerebellar artery
- Anterior inferior cerebellar artery
- Posterior inferior cerebellar artery

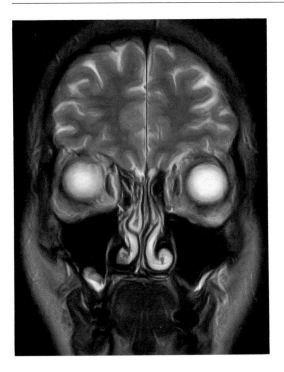

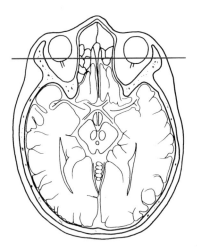

■ Frontal lobe

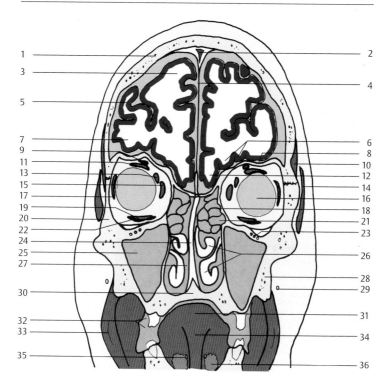

1 Frontal bone
2 Superior sagittal sinus
3 Superior frontal gyrus
4 Falx cerebri
5 Middle frontal gyrus
6 Orbital gyri
7 Superior frontal gyrus
8 Orbital roof
9 Levator palpebrae superioris muscle
10 Temporalis muscle
11 Superior rectus muscle
12 Gyrus rectus
13 Superior oblique muscle
14 Orbicularis oculi muscle
15 Medial rectus muscle
16 Eyeball
17 Lateral rectus muscle
18 Orbital plate of ethmoid bone
19 Inferior rectus muscle

20 Zygomatic bone
21 Ethmoid labyrinth
22 Inferior oblique muscle
23 Infraorbital artery, vein and nerve
24 Nasal septum
25 Maxillary sinus
26 Nasal turbinates (middle and inferior)
27 Nasal cavity
28 Maxilla
29 Parotid duct
30 Hard palate
31 Tongue
32 Oral cavity
33 Depressor anguli oris muscle
34 Genioglossus muscle
35 Submandibular duct
36 Sublingual gland

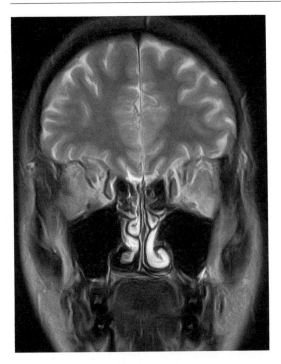

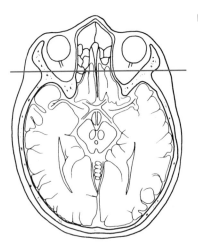

▨ Frontal lobe

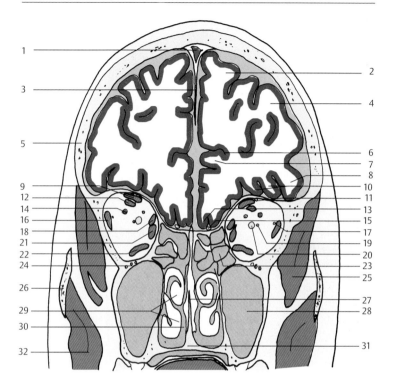

1   Superior sagittal sinus
2   Superior frontal gyrus
3   Falx cerebri
4   Middle frontal gyrus
5   Frontal bone
6   Cingulate sulcus
7   Cingulate gyrus
8   Inferior frontal gyrus
9   Levator palpebrae superioris muscle
10 Orbital gyri
11 Trochlear nerve
12 Superior rectus muscle
13 Gyrus rectus
14 Superior ophthalmic vein
15 Olfactory tract
16 Lateral rectus muscle
17 Abducens nerve
18 Superior oblique muscle
19 Ophthalmic artery
20 Optic nerve
21 Medial rectus muscle
22 Inferior rectus muscle
23 Ethmoid labyrinth
24 Infraorbital nerve, artery and vein
25 Temporalis muscle
26 Zygomatic arch
27 Nasal septum
28 Maxillary sinus
29 Nasal turbinates (middle and inferior)
30 Nasal cavity
31 Hard palate
32 Masseter muscle

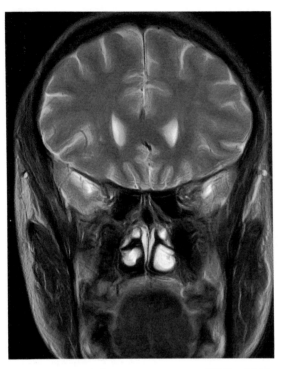

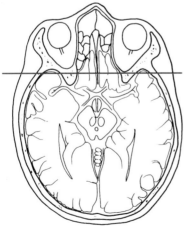

Frontal lobe
Temporal lobe

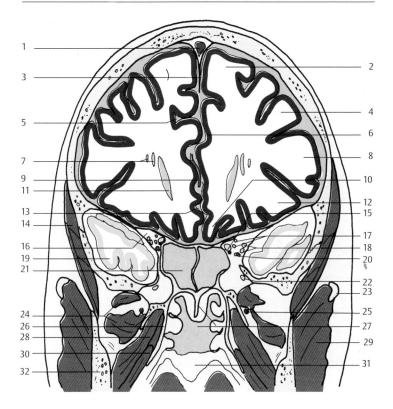

1 Superior sagittal sinus
2 Superior frontal gyrus
3 Falx cerebri
4 Middle frontal gyrus
5 Cingulate sulcus
6 Cingulate gyrus
7 Lentiform nucleus
8 Inferior frontal gyrus
9 Anterior cerebral artery
10 Gyrus rectus
11 Lateral ventricle (frontal horn)
12 Orbital gyrus
13 Anterior longitudinal fissure
14 Temporalis muscle
15 Optic nerve (cranial nerve II)
16 Superior orbital fissure
17 Trochlear and oculomotor nerves (cranial nerves IV and III)
18 Ophthalmic nerve (first division of trigeminal) and abducens nerve (cranial nerve VI)
19 Temporal lobe (anterior pole)
20 Ophthalmic artery and vein
21 Sphenoid sinus
22 Maxillary nerve (second division of trigeminal)
23 Zygomatic arch
24 Lateral pterygoid muscle
25 Maxillary artery
26 Pterygoid process (lateral and medial plates)
27 Nasal cavity and septum
28 Medial pterygoid muscle
29 Masseter muscle
30 Tensor veli palatini muscle
31 Soft palate
32 Mandible (ramus)

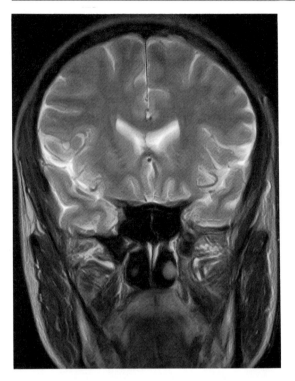

Frontal lobe
Temporal lobe

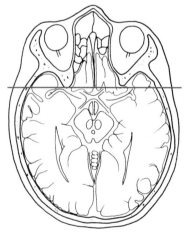

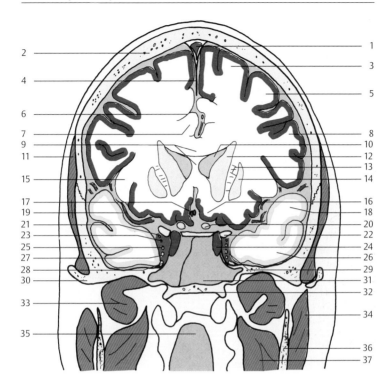

1 Superior sagittal sinus	**21** Oculomotor nerve (cranial nerve III)
2 Parietal bone	**22** Anterior clinoid process
3 Superior frontal gyrus	**23** Trochlear nerve (cranial nerve IV)
4 Falx cerebri	**24** Internal carotid artery
5 Middle frontal gyrus	**25** Ophthalmic nerve (first division of trigeminal)
6 Cingulate sulcus	
7 Cingulate gyrus	**26** Middle temporal gyrus
8 Inferior frontal gyrus	**27** Abducens nerve (cranial nerve VI)
9 Corpus callosum (genu)	**28** Maxillary nerve (second division of trigeminal)
10 Lateral ventricle (anterior horn)	
11 Temporalis muscle	**29** Cavernous sinus
12 Caudate nucleus (head)	**30** Zygomatic arch
13 Internal capsule	**31** Sphenoid sinus
14 Putamen	**32** Sphenoid bone
15 Insula	**33** Lateral pterygoid muscle
16 Gyrus rectus	**34** Masseter muscle
17 Anterior cerebral artery	**35** Nasopharynx
18 Superior temporal gyrus	**36** Mandible (ramus)
19 Insular arteries	**37** Medial pterygoid muscle
20 Optic nerve (cranial nerve II)	

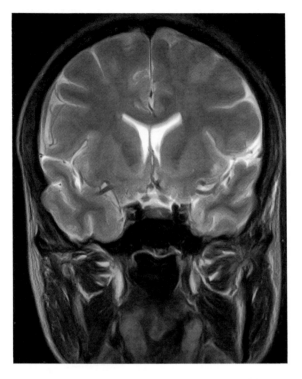

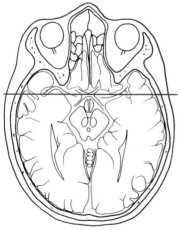

▨ Frontal lobe
▢ Temporal lobe

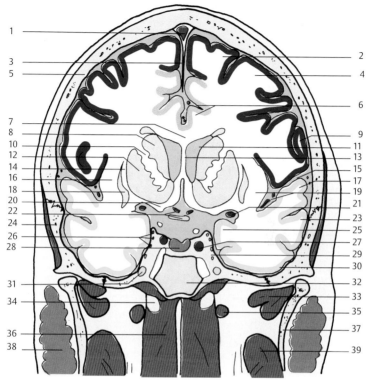

1   Superior sagittal sinus
2   Superior frontal gyrus
3   Falx cerebri
4   Middle frontal gyrus
5   Parietal bone
6   Cingulate sulcus and gyrus
7   Corpus callosum (trunk)
8   Caudate nucleus (head)
9   Inferior frontal gyrus
10 Internal capsule (anterior limb)
11 Lateral ventricle (anterior horn)
12 Putamen
13 Septum pellucidum
14 External capsule
15 Lateral sulcus
16 Capsula extrema
17 Superior temporal gyrus
18 Claustrum
19 Insula and insular cistern
20 Roof of chiasmatic cistern and olfactory tract
21 Middle cerebral artery
22 Optic chiasm and anterior cerebral artery
23 Middle temporal gyrus
24 Temporal bone
25 Parahippocampal gyrus
26 Oculomotor, trochlear and abducens nerves (cranial nerves III, IV, VI)
27 Internal carotid artery
28 Pituitary
29 Cavernous sinus
30 Lateral occipitotemporal gyrus
31 Trigeminal (gasserian) ganglion
32 Sphenoid sinus
33 Lateral pterygoid muscle
34 Eustachian tube
35 Levator veli palatini muscle
36 Nasopharynx
37 Mandible (ramus)
38 Parotid gland
39 Medial pterygoid muscle

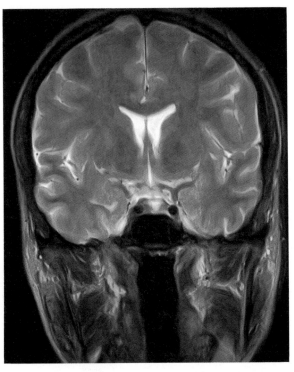

■ Frontal lobe
☐ Temporal lobe

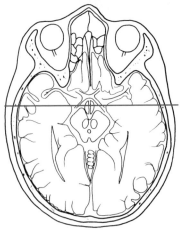

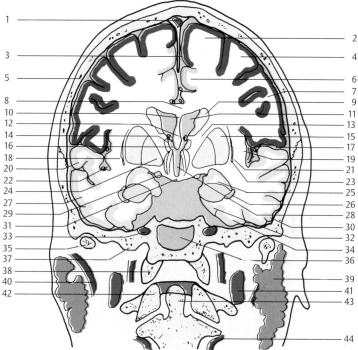

1	Superior sagittal sinus	**23**	External capsule
2	Superior frontal gyrus	**24**	Globus pallidus
3	Falx cerebri	**25**	Amygdaloid body
4	Middle frontal gyrus	**26**	Lateral ventricle (temporal horn)
5	Parietal bone	**27**	Middle temporal gyrus
6	Cingulate gyrus	**28**	Third ventricle
7	Precentral gyrus	**29**	Optic tract
8	Corpus callosum (trunk)	**30**	Inferior temporal gyrus
9	Caudate nucleus (body)	**31**	Mamillary body
10	Septum pellucidum	**32**	Parahippocampal gyrus
11	Lateral ventricle	**33**	Internal carotid artery
12	Fornix	**34**	Lateral occipitotemporal gyrus
13	Internal capsule	**35**	Mandibular condyle
14	Thalamus (anterior nuclei)	**36**	Sphenoid sinus
15	Putamen	**37**	Sphenoid bone
16	Interventricular foramen (of Monro)	**38**	Occipital condyle
17	Lateral sulcus	**39**	Parotid gland
18	Capsula extrema	**40**	External carotid artery
19	Insula	**41**	Internal jugular vein
20	Superior temporal gyrus	**42**	Atlas (lateral mass)
21	Claustrum	**43**	Dens of axis
22	Insular cistern	**44**	Vertebral artery

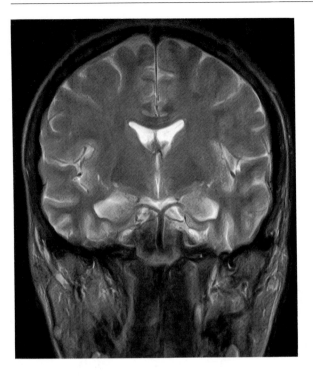

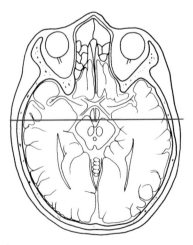

■ Frontal lobe
☐ Temporal lobe
■ Parietal lobe
■ Pons

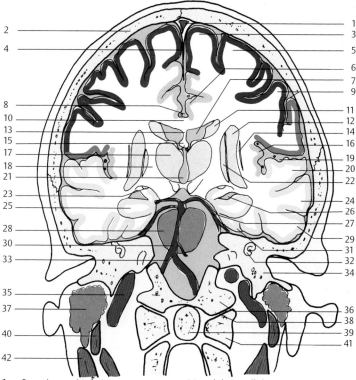

1	Superior sagittal sinus	**22**	Globus pallidus
2	Parietal bone	**23**	Optic tract
3	Superior frontal gyrus	**24**	Middle temporal gyrus
4	Falx cerebri	**25**	Hippocampus
5	Middle frontal gyrus	**26**	Lateral ventricle (temporal horn)
6	Cingulate gyrus	**27**	Posterior cerebral artery
7	Lateral ventricle	**28**	Pons
8	Pericallosal artery	**29**	Inferior temporal gyrus
9	Precentral gyrus, central sulcus	**30**	Basilar artery
10	Corpus callosum (trunk)	**31**	Parahippocampal gyrus
11	Caudate nucleus (head)	**32**	Cochlea
12	Putamen	**33**	Vertebral artery
13	Septum pellucidum	**34**	Temporal bone
14	Claustrum	**35**	Internal jugular vein
15	Fornix	**36**	Occipital condyle
16	Insula	**37**	Parotid gland
17	Thalamus	**38**	Atlantooccipital joint
18	Internal capsule	**39**	Dens of axis
19	Lateral sulcus	**40**	Digastric muscle (posterior belly)
20	Superior temporal gyrus	**41**	Atlas (lateral mass)
21	Third ventricle	**42**	Sternocleidomastoid muscle

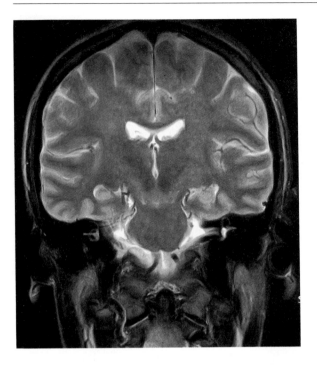

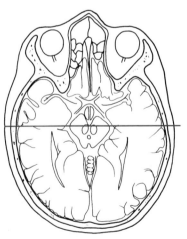

- ■ Frontal lobe
- □ Temporal lobe
- ■ Parietal lobe
- □ Mesencephalon
- ▨ Pons
- ■ Medulla oblongata

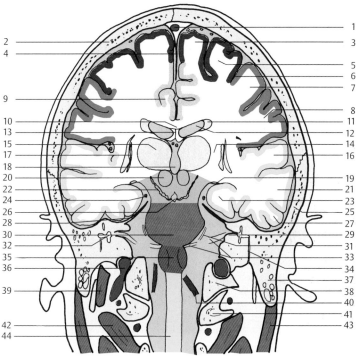

1 Superior sagittal sinus	**23** Parahippocampal gyrus
2 Parietal bone	**24** Posterior cerebral artery
3 Superior frontal gyrus	**25** Temporal bone
4 Falx cerebri	**26** Interpeduncular cistern
5 Precentral gyrus	**27** Inferior temporal gyrus
6 Central sulcus	**28** Tentorium of cerebellum
7 Postcentral gyrus	**29** Internal auditory canal
8 Supramarginal gyrus	**30** Pons
9 Cingulate gyrus	**31** Trigeminal nerve
10 Corpus callosum (trunk)	**32** Cochlea
11 Caudate nucleus	**33** Vestibulocochlear nerve
12 Lateral ventricle	**34** Facial canal
13 Fornix	**35** Medulla oblongata
14 Internal capsule	**36** Internal jugular vein
15 Thalamus	**37** Mastoid process
16 Superior temporal gyrus	**38** Occipital condyle
17 Lentiform nucleus (putamen, globus pallidus)	**39** Digastric muscle
	40 Vertebral artery
18 Third ventricle	**41** Atlas (lateral mass)
19 Optic tract	**42** Obliquus capitis muscle
20 Red nucleus	**43** Sternocleidomastoid muscle
21 Middle temporal gyrus	**44** Spinal cord
22 Substantia nigra	

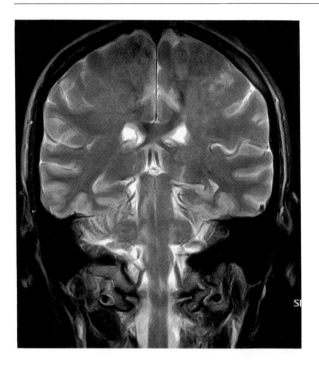

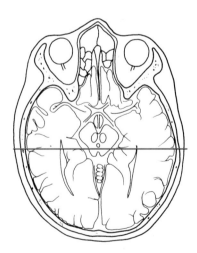

- ■ Frontal lobe
- □ Temporal lobe
- ▨ Parietal lobe
- ■ Cerebellum
- ▨ Mesencephalon
- ▨ Pons
- ■ Medulla oblongata

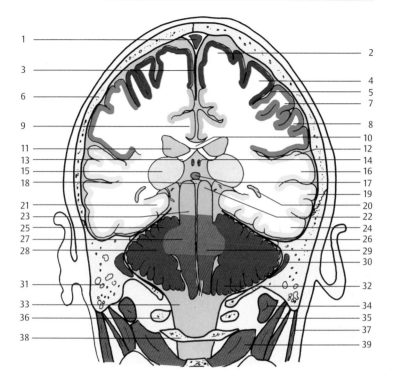

1	Superior sagittal sinus	**20**	Lateral ventricle (temporal horn)
2	Superior frontal gyrus	**21**	Parahippocampal gyrus
3	Falx cerebri	**22**	Cranial colliculus
4	Precentral gyrus	**23**	Mesencephalon
5	Central sulcus	**24**	Inferior temporal gyrus
6	Parietal bone	**25**	Cerebellum (cranial lobe)
7	Postcentral gyrus	**26**	Tentorium of cerebellum
8	Supramarginal gyrus	**27**	Roof of fourth ventricle
9	Cingulate gyrus	**28**	Middle cerebellar peduncle
10	Corpus callosum	**29**	Pons
11	Lateral ventricle	**30**	Sigmoid sinus
12	Transverse temporal gyrus (Heschl's gyrus)	**31**	Mastoid process
13	Fornix	**32**	Floccule
14	Internal cerebral vein	**33**	Cisterna magna
15	Thalamus	**34**	Obliquus capitis superior muscle
16	Superior temporal gyrus	**35**	Rectus capitis superior muscle
17	Pineal gland	**36**	Atlas (posterior arch)
18	Aqueduct (inlet)	**37**	Sternocleidomastoid muscle
19	Middle temporal gyrus	**38**	Axis (arch)
		39	Obliquus capitis inferior muscle

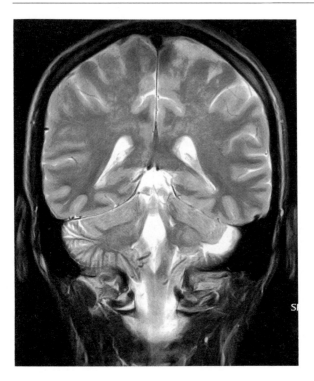

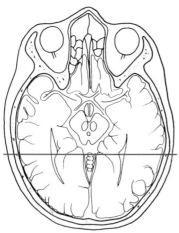

Frontal lobe
Temporal lobe
Parietal lobe
Cerebellum

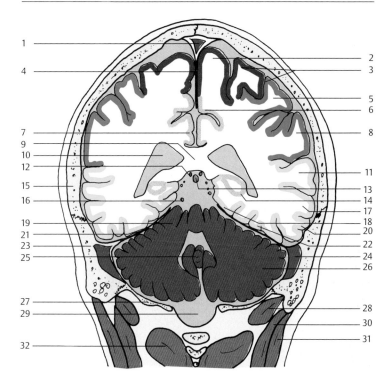

1 Superior sagittal sinus	**18** Medial occipitotemporal gyrus
2 Precentral gyrus	**19** Cerebellum (cranial lobe)
3 Precentral gyrus, central sulcus	**20** Inferior temporal gyrus
4 Falx cerebri	**21** Tentorium of cerebellum
5 Postcentral gyrus	**22** Lateral occipitotemporal gyrus
6 Paracentral lobule	**23** Temporal bone
7 Cingulate gyrus	**24** Sigmoid sinus
8 Supramarginal gyrus	**25** Uvula of cerebellum
9 Corpus callosum (splenium)	**26** Cerebellum (caudal lobe)
10 Lateral ventricle (trigone)	**27** Occipital bone
11 Superior temporal gyrus	**28** Obliquus capitis superior muscle
12 Internal cerebral vein	**29** Cisterna magna (cerebello-medullary cistern)
13 Pineal gland	**30** Longissimus capitis muscle
14 Hippocampus	**31** Splenius capitis muscle
15 Parietal bone	**32** Obliquus capitis inferior muscle
16 Superior cerebellar artery	
17 Middle temporal gyrus	

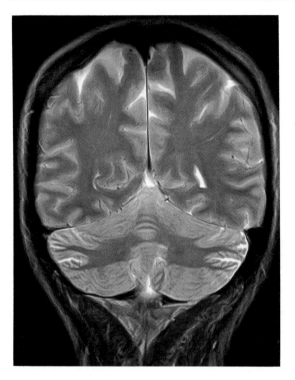

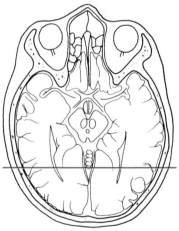

- ■ Frontal lobe
- □ Temporal lobe
- ▨ Parietal lobe
- ▨ Cerebellum

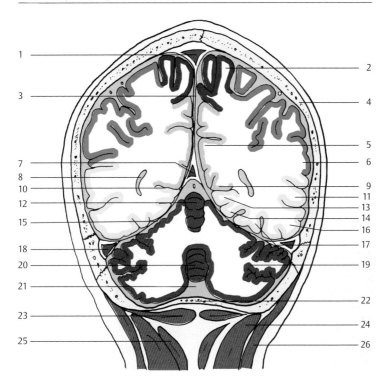

1 Superior sagittal sinus	**16** Inferior temporal gyrus
2 Precentral gyrus	**17** Lateral occipitotemporal gyrus
3 Falx cerebri	**18** Transverse sinus
4 Parietal bone	**19** Cerebellum (caudal lobe)
5 Precuneus	**20** Pyramid of vermis
6 Angular gyrus	**21** Cisterna magna (cerebellomedullary cistern)
7 Straight sinus	
8 Lateral ventricle (posterior horn)	**22** Occipital bone
9 Cuneus	**23** Rectus capitis posterior muscle (minor)
10 Calcarine sulcus	
11 Middle temporal gyrus	**24** Semispinalis capitis muscle
12 Cerebellum (cranial lobe)	**25** Rectus capitis posterior muscle (major)
13 Striate cortex	
14 Medial occipitotemporal gyrus	**26** Splenius capitis muscle
15 Tentorium of cerebellum	

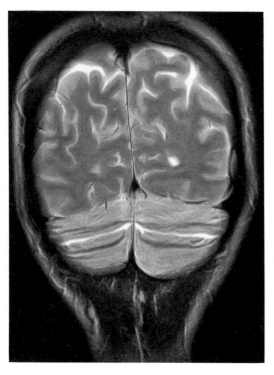

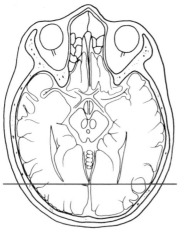

■ Parietal lobe
■ Occipital lobe
■ Cerebellum

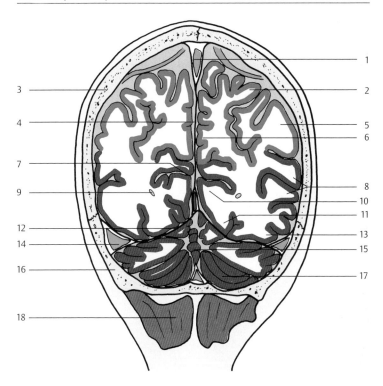

1 Superior sagittal sinus
2 Superior parietal lobule
3 Parietal bone
4 Falx cerebri
5 Angular gyrus
6 Precuneus
7 Calcarine sulcus
8 Occipital gyri
9 Lateral ventricle (posterior horn)
10 Cuneus
11 Medial occipitotemporal gyrus
12 Tentorium of cerebellum
13 Lateral occipitotemporal gyrus
14 Transverse sinus
15 Vermis of cerebellum
16 Occipital bone
17 Cerebellum (caudal lobe)
18 Semispinalis capitis muscle

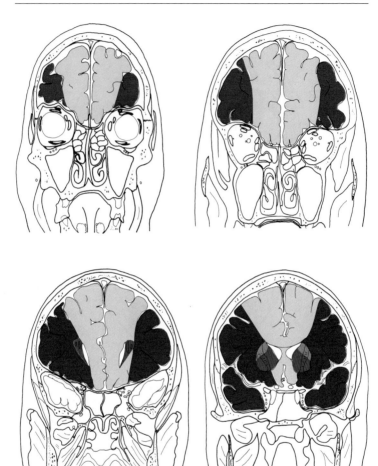

Anterior cerebral artery
- Terminal branches
- Central branches

Middle cerebral artery
- Terminal branches
- Central branches

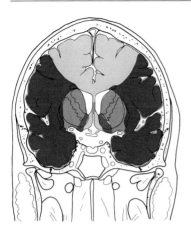

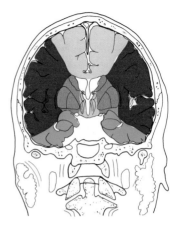

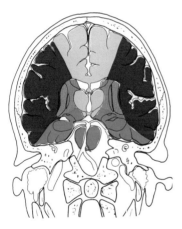

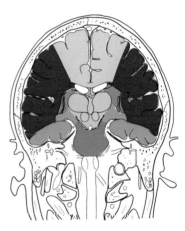

Anterior cerebral artery
☐ Terminal branches
■ Central branches

Middle cerebral artery
■ Terminal branches
▨ Central branches

Posterior cerebral artery
■ Terminal branches
☐ Central branches
■ Paramedian and circumferential
　arteries

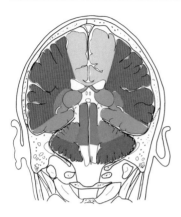
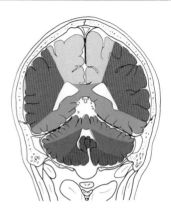
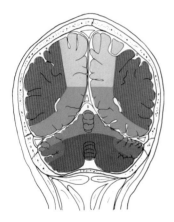
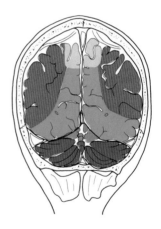

Anterior cerebral artery

☐ Terminal branches
■ Central branches

Middle cerebral artery

■ Terminal branches
▦ Central branches

Posterior cerebral artery

▨ Terminal branches
☐ Central branches

▧ Superior cerebellar artery
▦ Anterior inferior cerebellar artery
▨ Posterior inferior cerebellar artery
▨ Paramedian and circumferential
   arteries

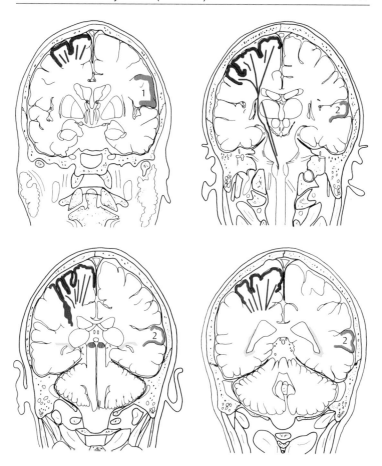

■ Motor system

Sensory system
■ Medial lemniscal tract
☐ Spinothalamic tract
■ Mesencephalic nucleus of trigeminal nerve

▨ Oculomotor nucleus and pathways
☐ Optic tract
▨ Speech center (1 = motor, 2 = sensory)

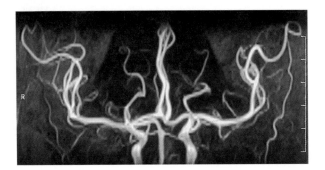

Frontal view

Anterior cerebral artery
Middle cerebral artery
Posterior cerebral artery

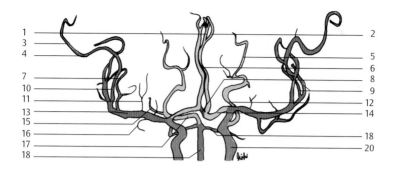

1 Callosomarginal artery
2 Pericallosal artery
3 Superior parietal artery
4 Middle cerebral artery
   (opercular part)
5 Parietooccipital artery
6 Anterior cerebral artery
   (postcommunicating part)
7 Insular arteries
8 Anterior communicating artery
9 Temporal artery
   (anterior and middle)
10 Middle cerebral artery (insular part)
11 Central branches of middle
   cerebral artery

12 Left posterior cerebral artery
   (from internal carotid artery,
   variant)
13 Middle cerebral artery
   (sphenoidal part)
14 Anterior cerebral artery
   (precommunicating part)
15 Temporooccipital artery
16 Temporal artery (from middle
   cerebral artery)
17 Right posterior cerebral artery
18 Superior cerebellar artery
19 Basilar artery
20 Internal carotid artery

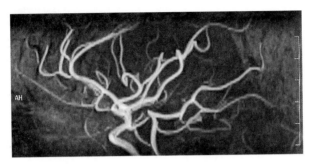

Lateral view

□ Anterior cerebral artery
▨ Middle cerebral artery
□ Posterior cerebral artery

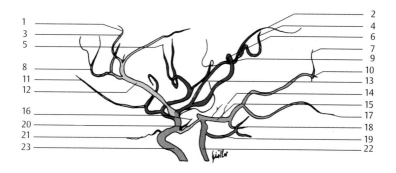

1 Callosomarginal artery
2 Parietal artery
3 Pericallosal artery
4 Artery of angular gyrus
5 Artery of precentral sulcus
   (prerolandic artery)
6 Middle cerebral artery
   (opercular part)
7 Parietooccipital artery
8 Frontopolar artery
9 Artery of central sulcus
   (rolandic artery)
10 Calcarine artery
11 Frontobasal artery

12 Anterior cerebral artery
    (segment 2)
13 Middle cerebral artery
    (segment 2)
14 Central arteries
15 Posterior cerebral artery
16 Anterior choroidal artery
17 Temporooccipital artery
18 Posterior temporal artery
19 Superior cerebellar artery
20 Posterior communicating artery
21 Ophthalmic artery
22 Basilar artery
23 Internal carotid artery

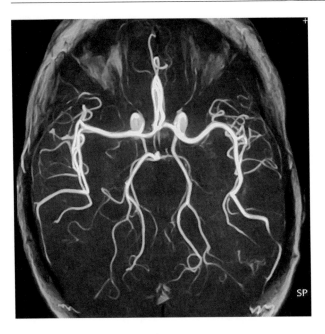

Superior view
- Anterior cerebral artery
- Middle cerebral artery
- Posterior cerebral artery

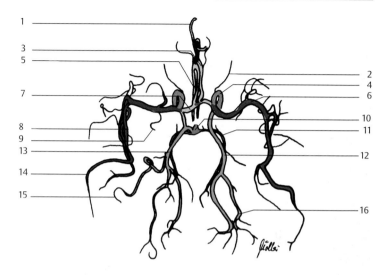

1 Frontal branch of anterior
   cerebral artery
2 Orbital branch
3 Anterior cerebral artery
   (postcommunicating part)
4 Internal carotid artery
5 Anterior communicating artery
6 Middle cerebral artery
   (sphenoidal part)
7 Anterior cerebral artery
   (precommunicating part)
8 Middle cerebral artery (insular part)
9 Anterior choroidal artery
10 Basilar artery
11 Superior cerebellar artery
12 Left posterior cerebral artery
   (from internal carotid artery,
   variant)
13 Right posterior cerebral artery
14 Middle cerebral artery
   (opercular part)
15 Temporal artery
16 Parietooccipital artery

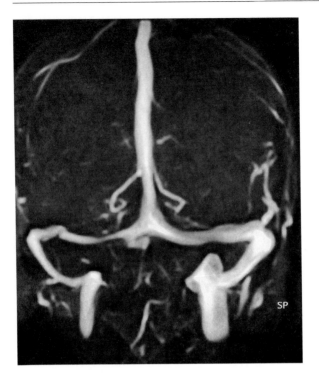

Frontal view

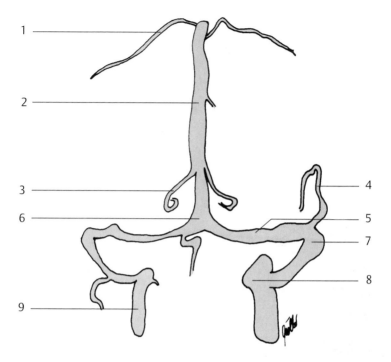

1 Parietal vein (of Rolando)
2 Superior sagittal sinus
3 Basal vein
4 Sphenoparietal sinus
5 Transverse sinus
6 Sinus confluence
7 Sigmoid sinus
8 Jugular bulb
9 Internal jugular vein

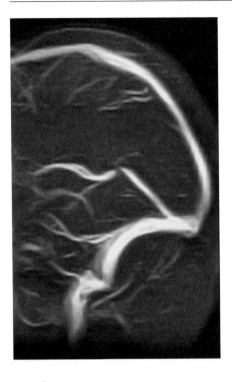

Lateral view

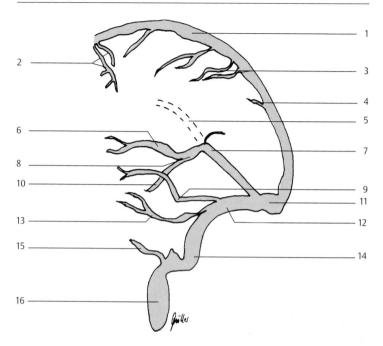

1 Superior sagittal sinus
2 Precentral veins
3 Parietal vein
4 Occipital veins
5 Inferior sagittal sinus
   (not visualized)
6 Internal cerebral vein
7 Straight sinus
8 Great cerebral vein

9 Inferior anastomotic vein
   (of Labbé)
10 Basal vein
11 Sinus confluence
12 Transverse sinus
13 Superior petrosal sinus
14 Sigmoid sinus
15 Inferior petrosal sinus
16 Internal jugular vein

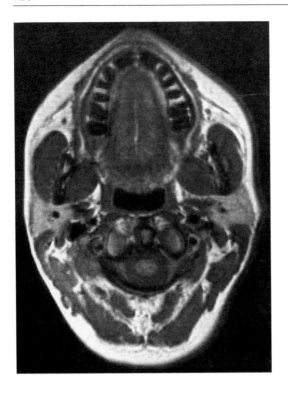

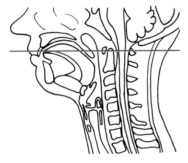

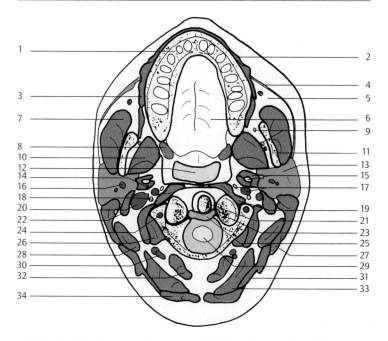

1 Maxilla (alveolar process)
2 Orbicularis oris muscle
3 Depressor anguli oris muscle
4 Parotid duct
5 Retromolar fossa
6 Hard palate
7 Masseter muscle
8 Palatine tonsil, superior pharyngeal constrictor muscle
9 Inferior alveolar nerve, lingual nerve
10 Medial pterygoid muscle
11 Mandible
12 Nasopharynx
13 Parotid gland
14 Cranial nerve XI
15 Styloid process and styloid muscles
16 Retromandibular vein
17 Internal carotid artery and cranial nerve XII

18 Cranial nerves IX and X
19 Longus capitis muscle
20 Internal jugular vein
21 Dens of axis
22 Digastric muscle (posterior belly)
23 Atlas (lateral mass)
24 Vertebral artery
25 Cruciform ligament of atlas
26 Obliquus capitis inferior and superior muscles
27 Sternocleidomastoid muscle
28 Longissimus capitis muscle
29 Spinal cord
30 Deep cervical vein
31 Splenius capitis muscle
32 Rectus capitis posterior muscle (major)
33 Semispinalis capitis muscle
34 Trapezius muscle

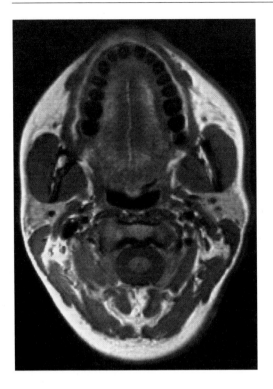

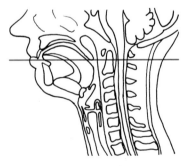

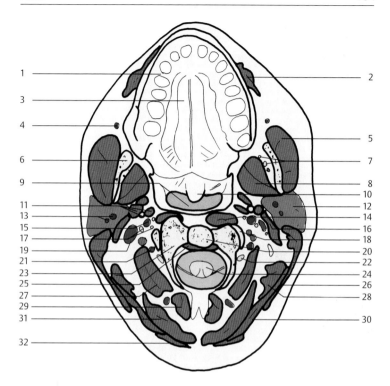

1	Maxilla (alveolar process)	17	Cranial nerves X and XII
2	Zygomaticus major muscle	18	Atlas (inferior arch)
3	Hard palate	19	Internal jugular vein
4	Facial artery	20	Dens of axis
5	Masseter muscle	21	Vertebral artery
6	Mandible (ramus)	22	Spinal nerve C2 (posterior root)
7	Lingual nerve and inferior alveolar nerve	23	Axis (body)
8	Medial pterygoid muscle	24	Spinal cord
9	Nasopharynx	25	Transverse ligament of atlas
10	Uvula and soft palate	26	Sternocleidomastoid muscle
11	Styloid process and styloid muscles	27	Inferior oblique muscle
12	Parotid gland	28	Longissimus capitis muscle
13	Superficial temporal artery and retromandibular vein	29	Rectus capitis posterior muscle (major)
14	Longus capitis muscle	30	Splenius capitis muscle
15	Internal carotid artery	31	Semispinalis capitis muscle
16	Digastric muscle (posterior belly)	32	Trapezius muscle

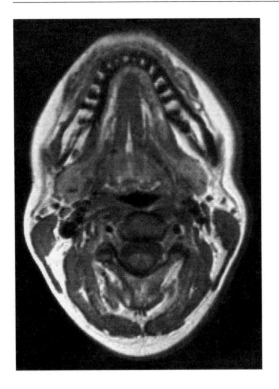

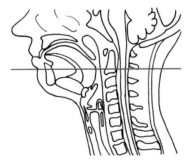

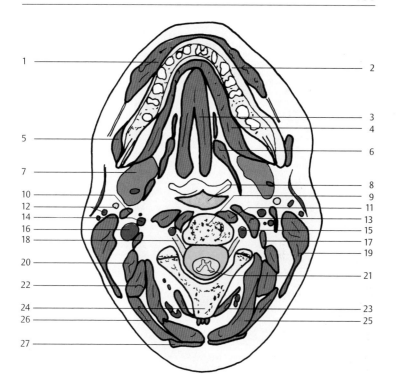

1 Depressor anguli oris muscle
2 Mandible (body)
3 Genioglossus muscle
4 Mylohyoid muscle
5 Masseter muscle
6 Hyoglossus muscle
7 Submandibular gland
8 Oropharynx
9 Axis (body)
10 Digastric muscle (posterior belly)
11 Longus colli muscle
12 Auriculotemporal nerve (branch) and retromandibular vein
13 Longus capitis muscle
14 Internal carotid artery
15 Vertebral artery
16 Internal jugular vein
17 Splenius cervicis muscle
18 Nerve root of C3
19 Sternocleidomastoid muscle
20 Levator scapulae muscle
21 Spinal cord (cervical)
22 Longissimus cervicis muscle
23 Inferior oblique muscle
24 Spinous process
25 Semispinalis capitis muscle
26 Splenius capitis muscle
27 Trapezius muscle

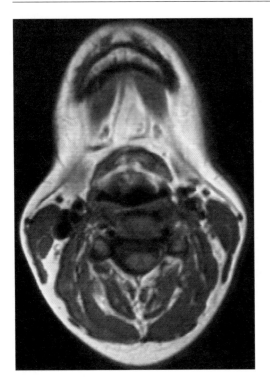

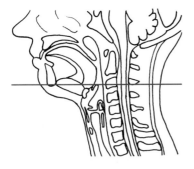

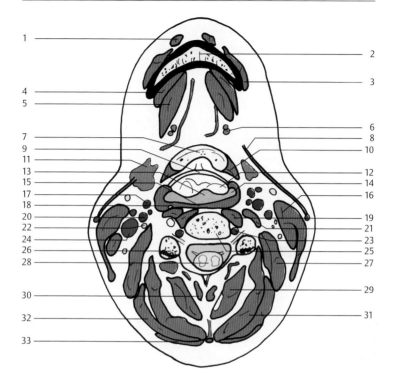

1 Mentalis muscle
2 Mandible
3 Depressor anguli oris muscle
4 Mylohyoid muscle
5 Geniohyoid muscle
6 Sublingual gland
7 Hyoid bone
8 Platysma
9 Epiglottis
10 Infrahyoid muscles
11 Submandibular gland
12 Aryepiglottic fold
13 Larynx
14 Piriform sinus
15 Inferior pharyngeal constrictor muscle and retropharyngeal space
16 Sternocleidomastoid muscle
17 External carotid artery
18 Sympathetic trunk
19 Longus colli muscle
20 Internal carotid artery
21 Anterior scalene muscle
22 Vagus nerve
23 Vertebral artery
24 Internal jugular vein
25 Body of C4 vertebra
26 C3/C4 facet joint
27 Levator scapulae and longissimus capitis muscles
28 Spinal cord (cervical)
29 Semispinalis cervicis muscle
30 Multifidus muscles
31 Semispinalis capitis muscle
32 Splenius capitis muscle
33 Trapezius muscle

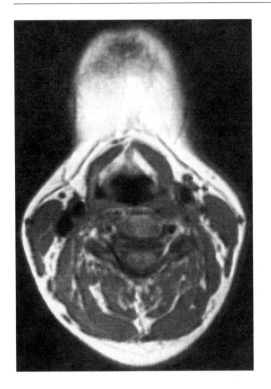

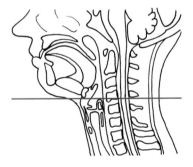

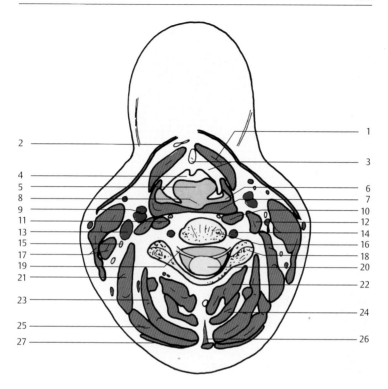

1 Infrahyoid muscles (sternohyoid
   and sternothyroid)
2 Platysma
3 Thyrohyoid membrane and
   preepiglottic space
4 Epiglottis
5 Larynx
6 Piriform sinus
7 Inferior pharyngeal constrictor
   muscle
8 Hypopharynx
9 Carotid artery (bifurcation)
10 Longus colli muscle
11 Sympathetic trunk
12 Anterior scalene muscle

13 Internal jugular vein
14 Vertebral artery
15 Vagus nerve
16 Body of C4 vertebra
17 Sternocleidomastoid muscle
18 C4/C5 facet joint
19 Spinal nerve
20 Spinal cord (cervical)
21 Levator scapulae muscle
22 Multifidus muscles
23 Semispinalis capitis muscle
24 Semispinalis cervicis muscle
25 Splenius capitis muscle
26 Nuchal ligament
27 Trapezius muscle

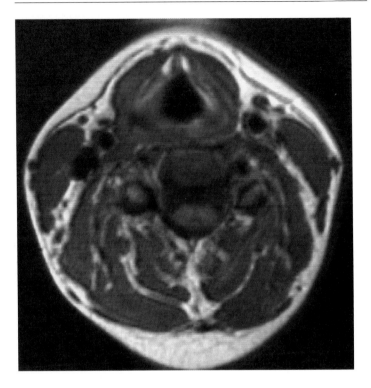

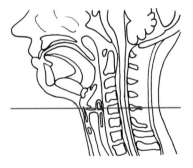

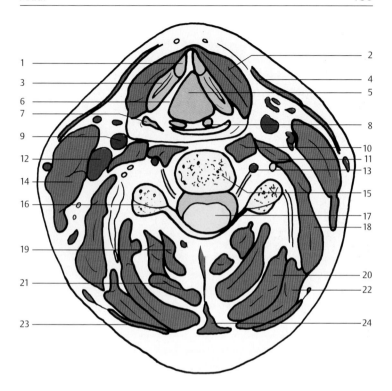

1 Thyroid cartilage (lamina)
2 Infrahyoid muscles (sternothyroid, omohyoid)
3 Thyroid cartilage
4 Platysma
5 Larynx (vestibule)
6 Vestibular fold
7 Piriform sinus
8 Arytenoid cartilage
9 Common carotid artery
10 Anterior scalene muscle
11 Longus colli muscle
12 Jugular vein
13 Vertebral artery
14 Sternocleidomastoid muscle
15 Body of C5 vertebra
16 C5/C6 facet joint
17 Spinal cord
18 Levator scapulae muscle
19 Multifidus muscles
20 Semispinalis capitis muscle
21 Semispinalis cervicis muscle
22 Splenius capitis muscle
23 Trapezius muscle
24 Nuchal ligament

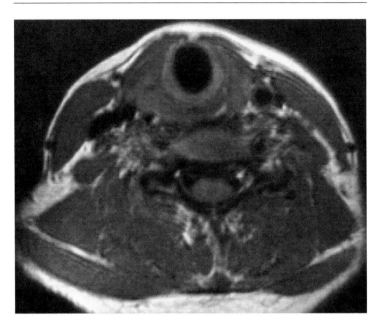

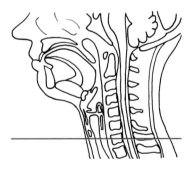

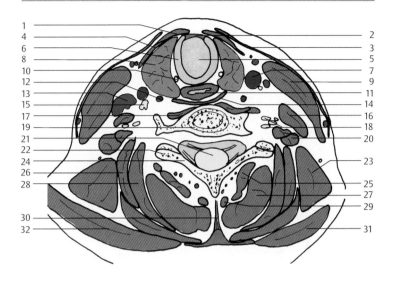

1 Sternohyoid muscle
2 Cricothyroid ligament
3 Platysma
4 Sternothyroid muscle
5 Infraglottic space
6 Cricoid cartilage
7 Common carotid artery
8 Thyroid gland
9 Sternocleidomastoid muscle
10 Thyroid cartilage, inferior cornu
11 Esophagus
12 Vertebral artery
13 Internal jugular vein
14 Inferior pharyngeal constrictor muscle
15 Vagus nerve
16 Anterior scalene muscle
17 Longus colli muscle
18 Brachial plexus
19 Body of C7 vertebra
20 Medial and posterior scalene muscles
21 Spinal cord (cervical)
22 Facet joint
23 Levator scapulae muscle
24 Arch of C7 vertebra
25 Multifidus muscles
26 Iliocostalis cervicis muscle
27 Semispinalis muscle
28 Longissimus muscle
29 Spinalis muscle
30 Nuchal ligament
31 Splenius cervicis and capitis muscles
32 Trapezius muscle

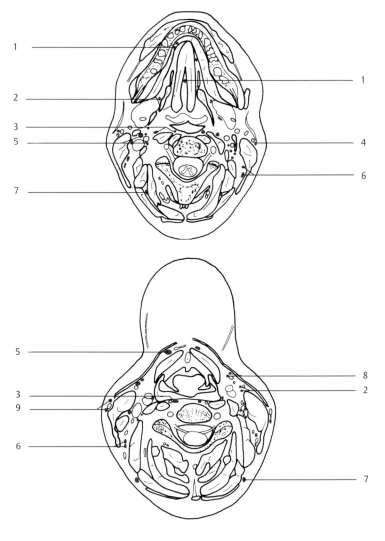

1 Submental lymph nodes
2 Submandibular lymph nodes
3 Retropharyngeal lymph nodes
4 Preauricular lymph nodes
5 Superior jugular group of nodes
6 Deep cervical lymph nodes
7 Nuchal lymph nodes
8 Anterior jugular lymph nodes
9 Superficial cervical lymph nodes

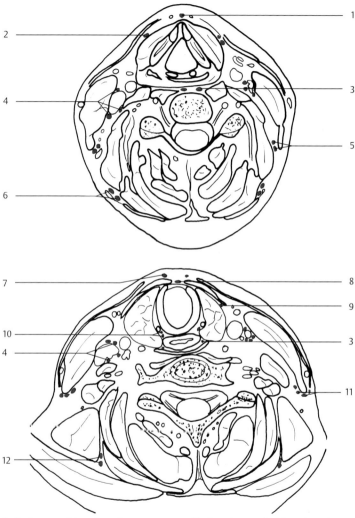

1 Prelaryngeal lymph nodes
2 Anterior jugular lymph nodes
3 Retropharyngeal lymph nodes
4 Inferior jugular group of nodes
5 Deep cervical lymph nodes
6 Nuchal lymph nodes
7 Anterior cervical lymph nodes
8 Pretracheal lymph nodes
9 Thyroid lymph nodes
10 Paratracheal lymph nodes
11 Supraclavicular lymph nodes
12 Superficial cervical lymph nodes

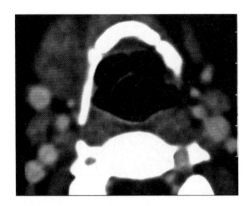

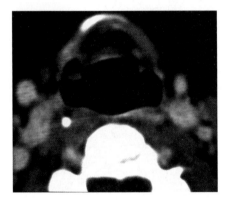

1

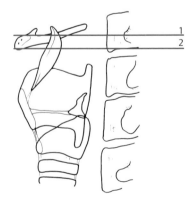

2

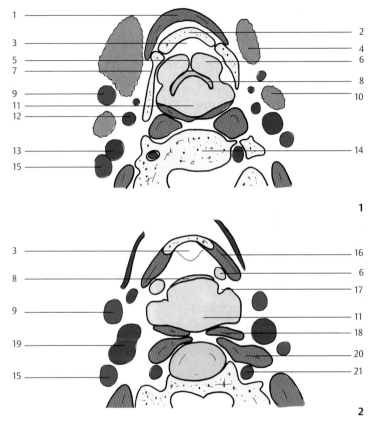

1 Infrahyoid muscles (mylohyoid, geniohyoid, hyoglossus)
2 Hyoid bone (body)
3 Preepiglottic space
4 Submandibular gland
5 Glossoepiglottic fold
6 Vallecula epiglottica
7 Hyoid bone (greater cornu)
8 Epiglottis
9 Anterior jugular vein
10 Parotid gland
11 Hypopharynx
12 External carotid artery
13 Internal carotid artery
14 Body of C3 vertebra
15 Internal jugular vein
16 Infrahyoid muscles (sternohyoid, sternothyroid)
17 Pharyngoepiglottic fold
18 Inferior pharyngeal constrictor muscle
19 Carotid bifurcation
20 Longus colli muscle
21 Vertebral artery

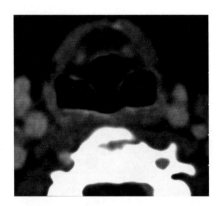

3

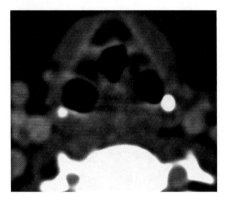

4

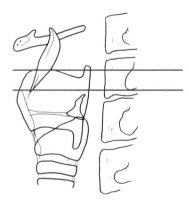

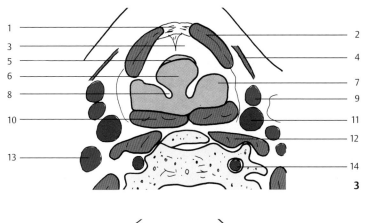

3

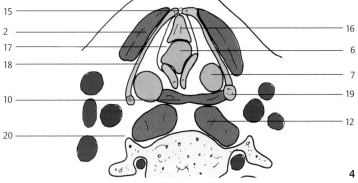

4

1 Thyrohyoid membrane	**11** Common carotid artery
2 Infrahyoid muscles (sternothyroid, omohyoid, thyrohyoid)	**12** Longus colli muscle
3 Preepiglottic space	**13** Internal jugular vein
4 Platysma	**14** Vertebral artery
5 Epiglottis	**15** Superior thyroid notch
6 Larynx	**16** Stem of epiglottis
7 Piriform sinus	**17** Vestibular folds
8 Aryepiglottic fold	**18** Thyroid cartilage (lamina)
9 Anterior jugular vein	**19** Thyroid cartilage (superior cornu)
10 Inferior pharyngeal constrictor muscle	**20** Body of C4 vertebra

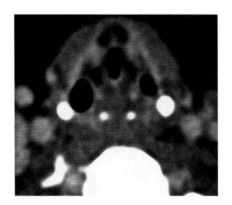

5

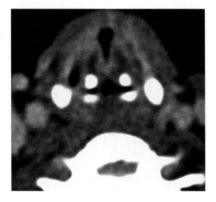

6

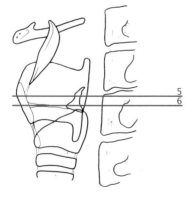

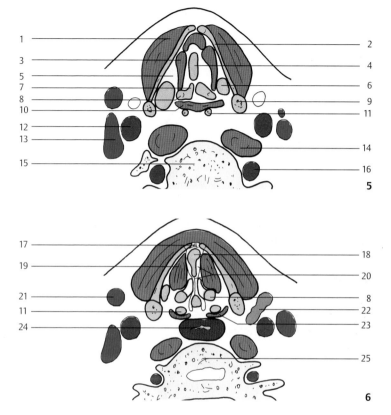

5

6

1	Infrahyoid muscles (sternothyroid, omohyoid, thyrohyoid)	**13**	Internal jugular vein
		14	Longus colli muscle
2	Thyroid cartilage	**15**	Body of C4 vertebra
3	Thyroarytenoid muscle	**16**	Vertebral artery
4	Larynx (vestibule)	**17**	Laryngeal prominence
5	Paralaryngeal space	**18**	Rima glottidis
6	Piriform sinus	**19**	Vocalis muscle
7	Arytenoid cartilage (vocal process)	**20**	Vocal cord
8	Arytenoid cartilage (body)	**21**	Anterior jugular vein
9	Thyroid cartilage (superior cornu)	**22**	Thyroid gland
10	Transverse arytenoid muscle	**23**	Oblique arytenoid muscle
11	Cricoid cartilage	**24**	Esophagus
12	Common carotid artery	**25**	Body of C5 vertebra

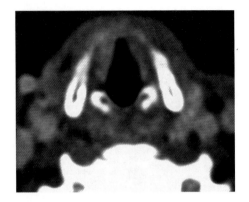

7

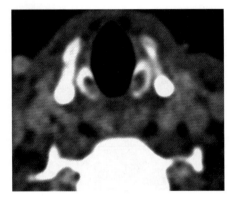

8

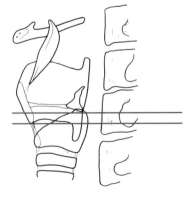

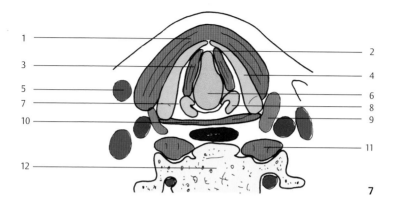

7

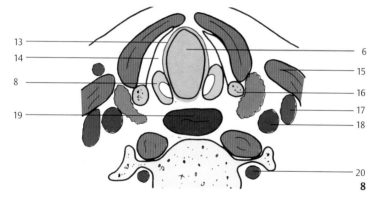

8

1 Infrahyoid muscles (sternohyoid, omohyoid, sternothyroid)
2 Anterior laryngeal commissure
3 Vocalis muscle
4 Thyroid cartilage
5 Anterior jugular vein
6 Subglottic space
7 Cricothyroid joint
8 Cricoid cartilage (lamina)
9 Thyroid gland
10 Inferior pharyngeal constrictor muscle

11 Longus colli muscle
12 Body of C6 vertebra
13 Conus elasticus
14 Paralaryngeal space
15 Sternocleidomastoid muscle
16 Thyroid cartilage (inferior cornu)
17 Internal jugular vein
18 Common carotid artery
19 Esophagus
20 Vertebral artery

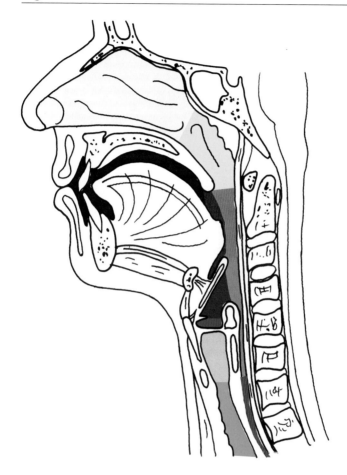

Nasal vestibule
(nasal cavity)
Nasopharynx

Oral cavity proper
Faucial isthmus
Oropharynx

Laryngeal part of pharynx
Esophagus
Laryngeal vestibule
Laryngeal ventricle
Infraglottic space
Trachea

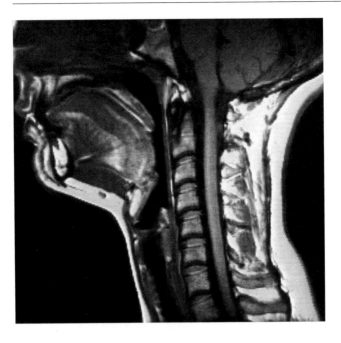

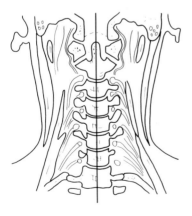

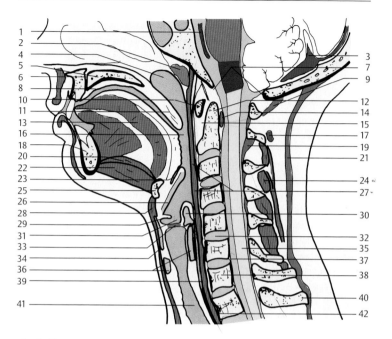

1 Basilar artery
2 Pharyngeal tonsil
3 Sinus confluence
4 Nasopharynx
5 Hard palate
6 Incisive fossa
7 Foramen magnum
8 Soft palate
9 Posterior atlantooccipital
  membrane
10 Atlas (anterior arch)
11 Uvula
12 Dens of axis
13 Genioglossus muscle
14 Transverse ligament of atlas
15 Retropharyngeal space
16 Oropharynx
17 Deep occipital veins
18 Mandible
19 Ligamenta flava
20 Geniohyoid muscle
21 Nuchal ligament
22 Mylohyoid muscle

23 Vallecula
24 Interspinal muscle
25 Hyoid bone
26 Epiglottis
27 Middle pharyngeal constrictor
  muscle
28 Sternohyoid and sternothyroid
  muscles
29 Vestibular fold
30 Arytenoid muscle
31 Larynx (vestibule)
32 Intervertebral disk space
33 Vocal cord
34 Thyroid cartilage
35 Spinal cord
36 Cricoid cartilage
37 Posterior longitudinal ligament
38 Body of C7 vertebra
39 Esophagus
40 Spinous process of C7 vertebra
41 Trachea
42 Anterior longitudinal ligament

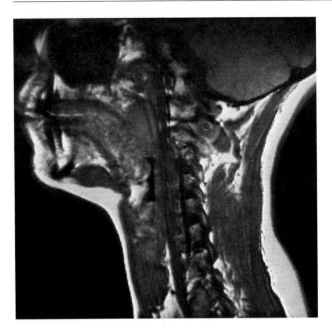

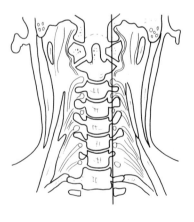

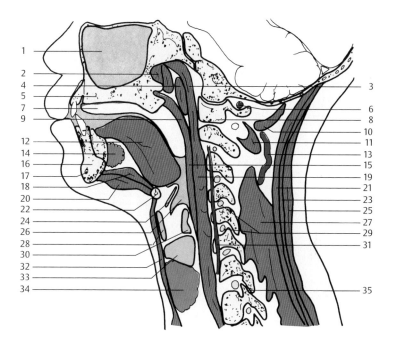

1 Maxillary sinus
2 Medial pterygoid muscle
3 Longus capitis muscle
4 Levator veli palatini muscle
5 Maxilla
6 Vertebral artery
7 Soft palate
8 Atlas
9 Buccinator muscle, superior
   pharyngeal constrictor muscle
10 Rectus capitis posterior muscle
   (major and minor)
11 Obliquus capitis inferior muscle
12 Genioglossus muscle
13 Deep cervical vein
14 Sublingual gland
15 Middle pharyngeal constrictor
   muscle
16 Mandible
17 Inferior alveolar artery

18 Mylohyoid muscle
19 Longus colli muscle
20 Digastric muscle (anterior belly)
21 Semispinalis capitis muscle
22 Hyoid bone
23 Splenius capitis muscle
24 Epiglottis
25 Trapezius muscle
26 Larynx
27 Semispinalis cervicis muscle
28 Thyroid cartilage
29 Nerve roots
30 Arytenoid cartilage
31 Vertebral artery
32 Sternohyoid and thyrohyoid
   muscles
33 Cricoid cartilage
34 Thyroid gland
35 Facet joint

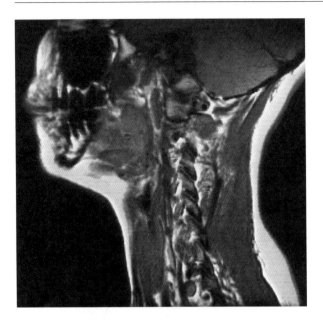

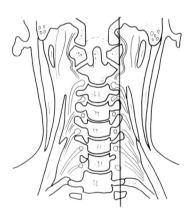

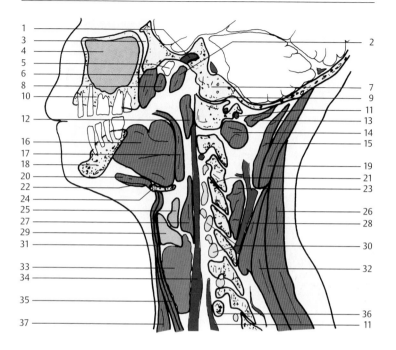

1 Internal carotid artery
2 Levator veli palatini muscle
3 Pterygopalatine fossa
4 Maxillary sinus
5 Eustachian tube
6 Medial pterygoid muscle
7 Occipital condyle
8 Tensor veli palatini muscle
9 Atlantooccipital articulation
10 Maxilla
11 Vertebral artery
12 Longus capitis muscle
13 Rectus capitis posterior muscle (major)
14 Obliquus capitis inferior muscle
15 Semispinalis capitis muscle
16 Tongue
17 Buccinator muscle and superior pharyngeal constrictor
18 Mandible
19 Splenius capitis muscle
20 Mylohyoid muscle
21 Facet joint
22 Digastric muscle (anterior belly)
23 Multifidus muscles
24 Hyoid bone
25 Piriform sinus
26 Trapezius muscle
27 Inferior pharyngeal constrictor muscle
28 Deep cervical vein
29 Thyroid cartilage
30 Nerve roots
31 Sternohyoid muscle
32 Semispinalis cervicis muscle
33 Thyroid gland
34 Common carotid artery
35 Sternothyroid muscle
36 First rib
37 Sternocleidomastoid muscle

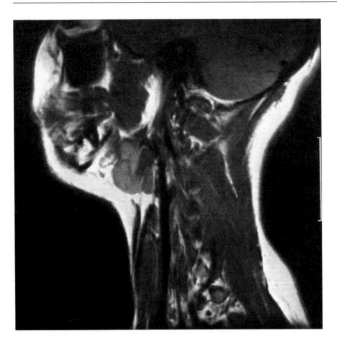

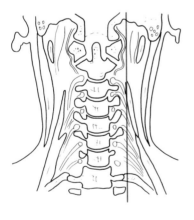

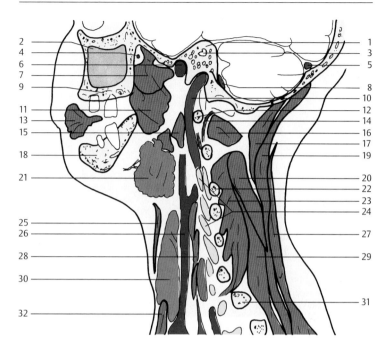

1 Petrous part of temporal bone
2 Maxillary sinus
3 Cochlea
4 Maxillary artery
5 Transverse sinus
6 Internal carotid artery
7 Lateral pterygoid muscle
8 Sigmoid sinus
9 Maxilla
10 Internal jugular vein
11 Medial pterygoid muscle
12 Atlas (transverse process)
13 Buccinator muscle
14 Vertebral artery
15 Stylopharyngeus muscle
16 Obliquus capitis inferior muscle
17 Semispinalis capitis muscle
18 Mandible
19 Splenius capitis muscle
20 Semispinalis cervicis muscle
21 Submandibular gland
22 Transverse process
23 Multifidus muscles
24 Cervical plexus
25 Platysma
26 Common carotid artery
27 Trapezius muscle
28 Longus colli muscle
29 Splenius cervicis muscle
30 Thyroid gland
31 Rib
32 Sternocleidomastoid muscle

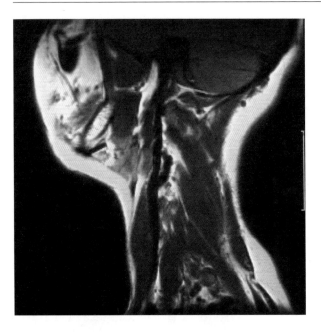

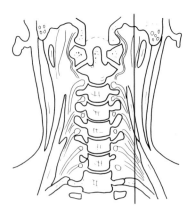

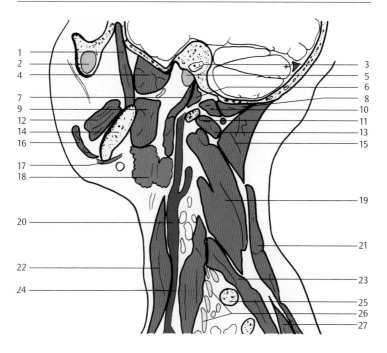

1   Temporalis muscle
2   Maxillary sinus
3   Mastoid antrum
4   Lateral pterygoid muscle
5   External auditory canal
6   Rectus capitis lateralis muscle
7   Stylopharyngeus muscle
8   Rectus capitis posterior muscle
    (major)
9   Medial pterygoid muscle
10 Obliquus capitis superior muscle
11 Atlas (transverse process)
12 Buccinator muscle
13 Obliquus capitis inferior muscle

14 Mandible
15 Splenius capitis muscle
16 Orbicularis oris muscle
17 Parotid duct
18 Submandibular gland
19 Multifidus muscles
20 Jugular vein
21 Trapezius muscle
22 Sternocleidomastoid muscle
23 Longissimus capitis muscle
24 Anterior scalene muscle
25 First rib
26 Cervical plexus
27 Levator scapulae muscle

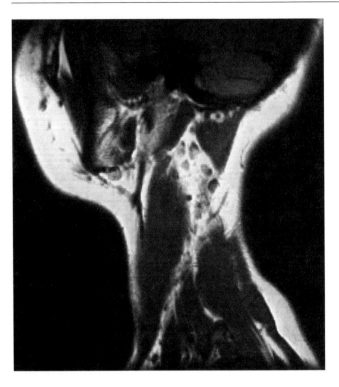

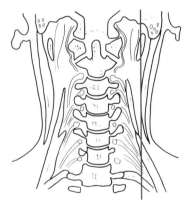

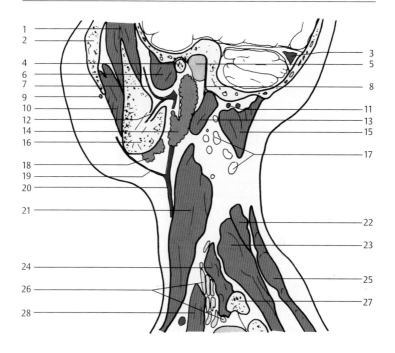

1 Temporalis muscle
2 Zygomatic bone
3 Transverse sinus
4 Temporomandibular joint
5 External auditory canal
6 Lateral pterygoid muscle
7 Maxillary artery
8 Facial nerve
9 Parotid duct
10 Masseter muscle
11 Suboccipital veins
12 Inferior alveolar artery
13 Digastric muscle (posterior belly)
14 Parotid gland

15 Splenius capitis muscle
16 Mandible
17 Lymph nodes
18 Submandibular gland
19 Facial artery
20 External carotid artery
21 Sternocleidomastoid muscle
22 Longissimus capitis muscle
23 Levator scapulae muscle
24 Medial scalene muscle
25 Trapezius muscle
26 Roots of brachial plexus
27 First rib
28 Anterior scalene muscle

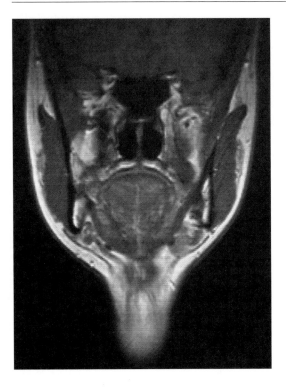

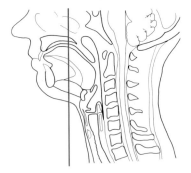

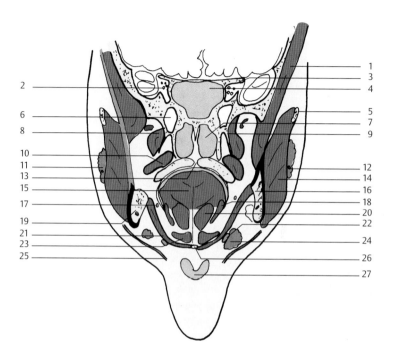

1 Temporalis muscle
2 Superior orbital fissure (with optic,
  trochlear, oculomotor, ophthalmic
  and abducens nerves)
3 Sphenoid bone
4 Sphenoid sinus
5 Zygomatic arch
6 Pterygopalatine fossa
7 Nasal cavity
8 Lateral pterygoid muscle
9 Pterygoid process
10 Medial pterygoid muscle
11 Parotid gland
12 Parotid duct
13 Soft palate
14 Masseter muscle
15 Tongue
16 Mandible (ramus)
17 Lingual nerve
18 Hyoglossus muscle
19 Mandibular canal (with inferior
   alveolar artery, nerve and vein)
20 Genioglossus muscle
21 Mylohyoid muscle
22 Digastric muscle (tendon)
23 Geniohyoid muscle
24 Submandibular gland
25 Platysma
26 Hyoid bone
27 Thyroid cartilage

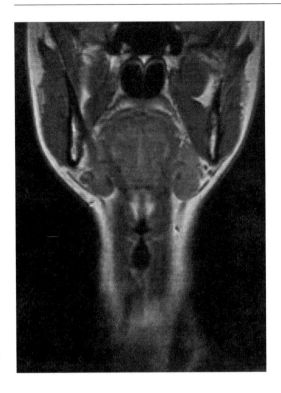

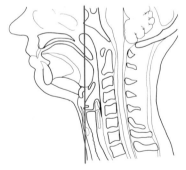

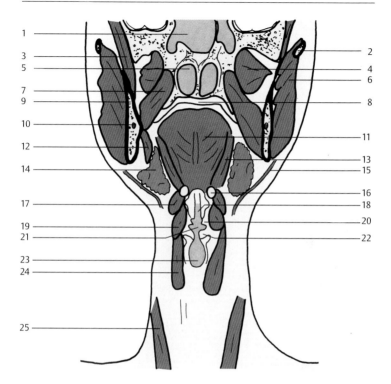

1 Sphenoid sinus
2 Zygomatic arch
3 Temporalis muscle
4 Lateral pterygoid muscle
5 Nasal cavity
6 Masseter muscle
7 Medial pterygoid muscle
8 Soft palate
9 Mandible (ramus)
10 Mandibular canal
11 Tongue
12 Mylohyoid muscle
13 Hyoglossus muscle
14 Submandibular gland
15 Platysma
16 Hyoid bone
17 Omohyoid muscle
18 Preepiglottic space
19 Thyrohyoid muscle
20 Vestibular ligament
21 Laryngeal ventricle
22 Vocal ligament
23 Infraglottic space
24 Sternohyoid muscle
25 Sternocleidomastoid muscle

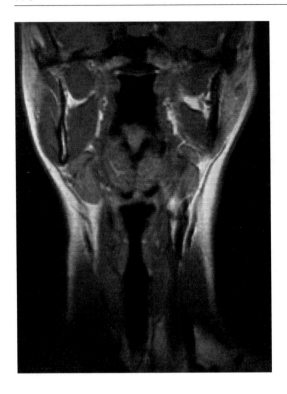

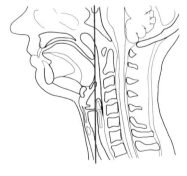

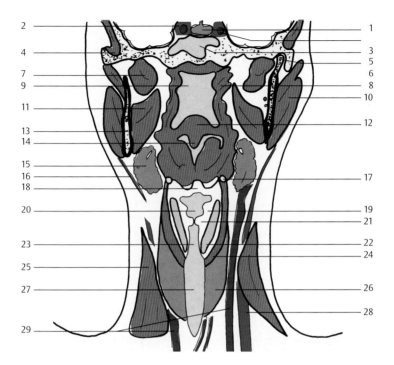

1 Pituitary
2 Cavernous sinus
3 Internal carotid artery
4 Temporalis muscle
5 Sphenoid sinus
6 Mandible (condyle)
7 Lateral pterygoid muscle
8 Pharyngeal musculature
9 Nasopharynx
10 Masseter muscle
11 Medial pterygoid muscle
12 Soft palate
13 Mandible (ramus)
14 Uvula
15 Submandibular gland

16 Platysma
17 Hyoid bone (greater cornu)
18 Epiglottis
19 Vestibular fold
20 Laryngeal vestibule
21 Vocal cord
22 Hyoid cartilage
23 Laryngeal cavity
24 Omohyoid, sternohyoid and
   thyrohyoid muscles
25 Sternocleidomastoid muscle
26 Thyroid gland
27 Trachea
28 Jugular vein
29 Common carotid artery

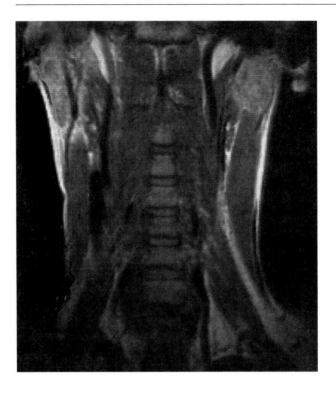

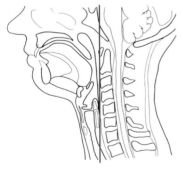

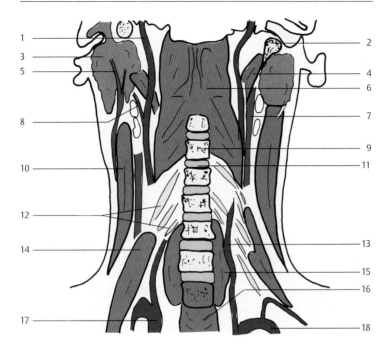

1 Internal carotid artery
2 Mandible (condyle)
3 Parotid gland
4 Lateral pterygoid muscle
5 Retromandibular vein
6 Pharyngeal constrictor muscle and longus capitis
7 Internal jugular vein
8 External carotid artery
9 Cervical vertebral body

10 Sternocleidomastoid muscle
11 Intervertebral disk
12 Cervical plexus
13 Vertebral artery
14 Anterior scalene muscle
15 Longissimus cervicis muscle
16 Esophagus
17 Brachiocephalic trunk
18 Subclavian artery

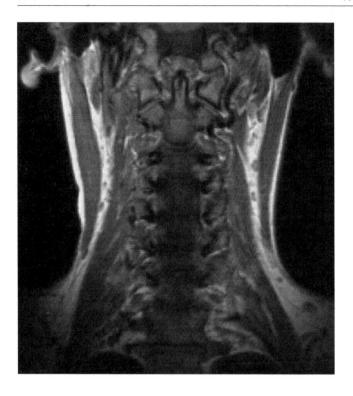

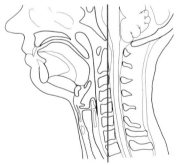

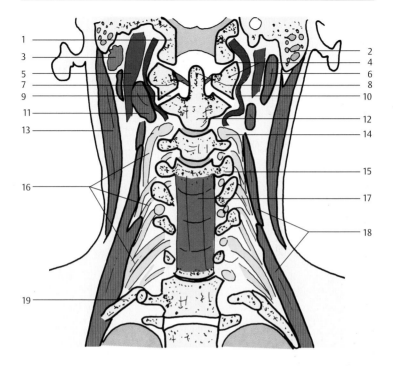

1 Occipital condyle
2 Mastoid process
3 Parotid gland
4 Atlas (lateral mass) and atlantooccipital articulation
5 Jugular vein
6 Digastric muscle
7 Alar ligaments
8 Dens of axis
9 Atlantoaxial articulation
10 Vertebral artery
11 Inferior oblique muscle
12 Axis
13 Sternocleidomastoid muscle
14 Root of nerve C3
15 Transverse process of C4 vertebra
16 Cervical plexus with nerve roots
17 Posterior longitudinal ligament (and cervical vertebrae)
18 Medial and posterior scalene muscles
19 First rib

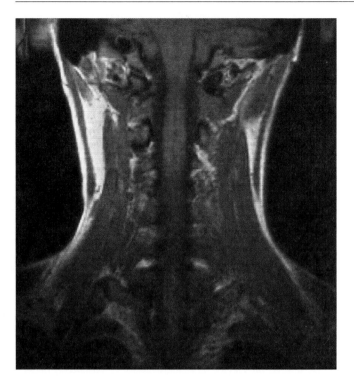

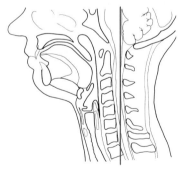

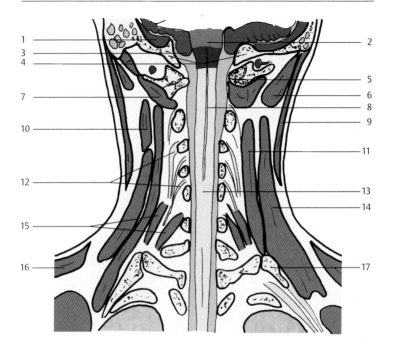

1 Sigmoid sinus
2 Medulla oblongata
3 Cerebellar fonsil
4 Foramen magnum
5 Atlas
6 Splenius cervicis muscle
7 Inferior oblique muscle
8 Median fissure (central canal)
9 Sternocleidomastoid muscle
10 Longissimus capitis muscle
11 Semispinalis cervicis muscle
12 Cervical plexus
13 Spinal cord
14 Levator scapulae muscle
15 Multifidus muscles
16 Trapezius muscle
17 First rib

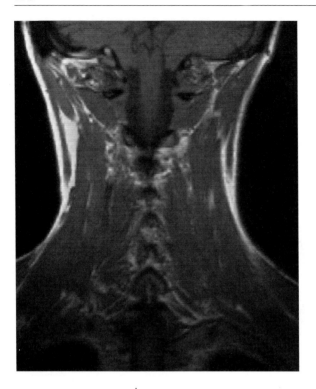

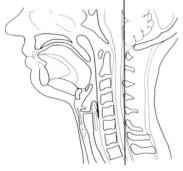

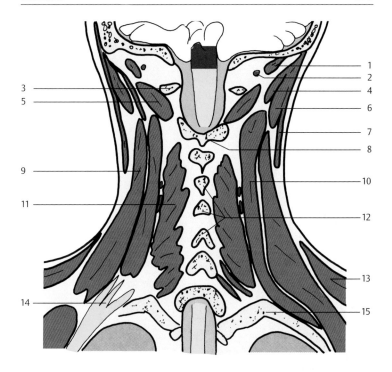

1   Obliquus capitis superior muscle
2   Deep cervical vein
3   Transverse process of C1 vertebra
4   Longissimus capitis muscle
5   Inferior oblique muscle
6   Splenius capitis muscle
7   Sternocleidomastoid muscle
8   Spinous process of axis
9   Levator scapulae muscle
10 Semispinalis muscle
11 Multifidus muscles
12 Spinous processes
    (of C4--C6 vertebrae)
13 Trapezius muscle
14 Cervical plexus
15 Rib

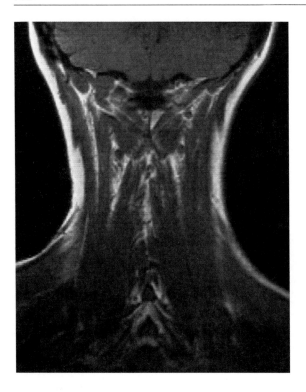

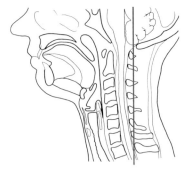

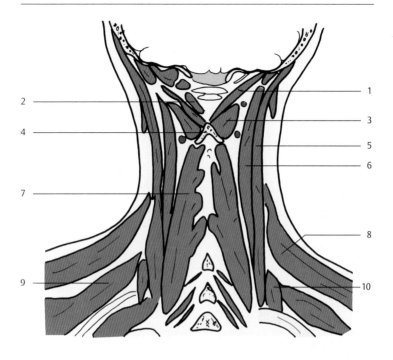

1 Rectus capitis posterior muscle (major)
2 Rectus capitis posterior muscle (minor)
3 Obliquus capitis inferior muscle
4 Spinous process of axis
5 Splenius capitis muscle
6 Semispinalis capitis muscle
7 Multifidus muscles
8 Trapezius muscle
9 Levator scapulae muscle
10 Rhomboid muscle

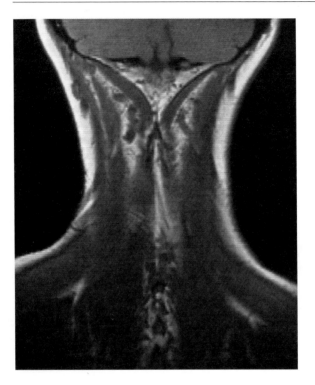

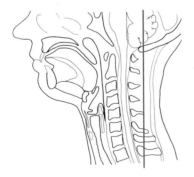

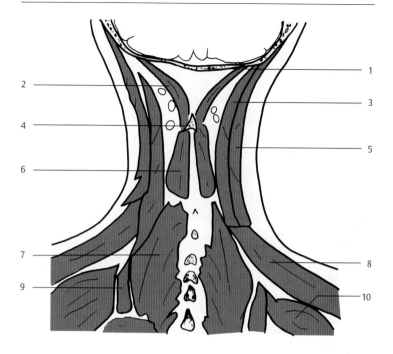

1 Occipital bone
2 Rectus capitis posterior muscle (major)
3 Semispinalis capitis muscle
4 Spinous process of axis
5 Splenius capitis muscle
6 Semispinalis cervicis muscle
7 Multifidus muscles
8 Trapezius muscle
9 Rhomboid muscle
10 Levator scapulae muscle

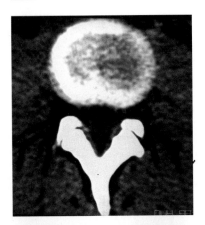

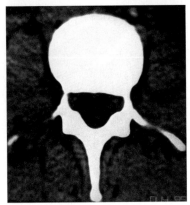

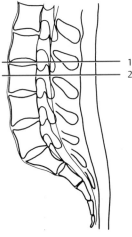

1
2

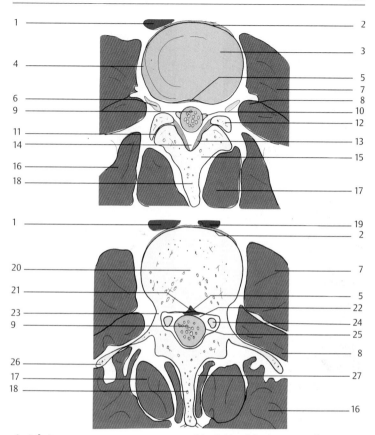

1 Inferior vena cava
2 Anterior longitudinal ligament
3 Intervertebral disk (L2/L3)
4 Anulus fibrosus
5 Posterior longitudinal ligament
6 Spinal nerve L2
7 Psoas muscle
8 Quadratus lumborum muscle
9 Cauda equina (in dural sac)
10 Spinal nerve L3 (emerging from dural sac)
11 Facet joint at L2/L3
12 Superior articular process (of L3 vertebra)
13 Ligamenta flava
14 Epidural fat (retrospinal trigone)
15 Inferior articular process (of L2 vertebra)
16 Erector spinae muscle
17 Multifidus muscles
18 Spinous process
19 Aorta (bifurcation)
20 Body of L3 vertebra
21 Basivertebral veins
22 Internal vertebral venous plexus
23 Pedicle
24 Nerve root
25 Dural sac
26 Transverse process
27 Paraspinal fat

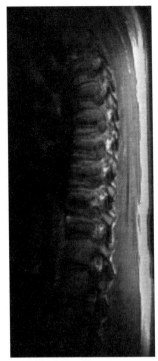

1

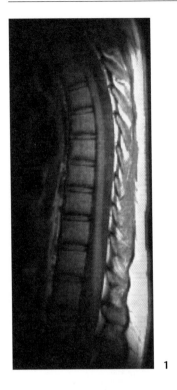

2

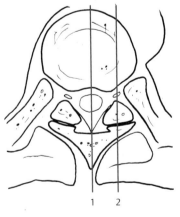

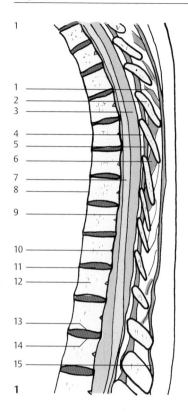
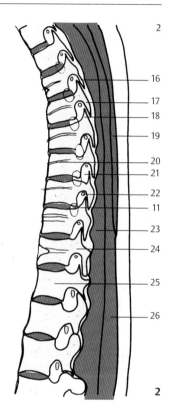

1 Supraspinal ligaments
2 Spinous process
3 Cerebrospinal fluid
  (postmedullary thecal space)
4 Epidural fat
5 Ligamenta flava
6 Interspinal ligaments
7 Spinal cord
8 Anterior longitudinal ligament
9 Posterior longitudinal ligament
10 Basivertebral veins
11 Intervertebral disk space
12 Thoracic vertebra
13 Inferior vertebral end plate

14 Superior vertebral end plate
15 Thoracolumbar fascia
16 Facet joints
17 Inferior articular process
18 Superior articular process
19 Trapezius muscle
20 Thoracic vessel
21 Intervertebral foramen
22 Nerve root
23 Multifidus muscles
24 Pedicle
25 Vertebral body
26 Erector spinae muscle

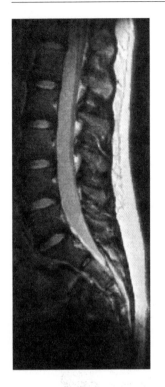

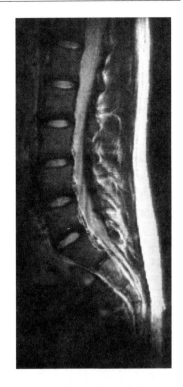

1

2

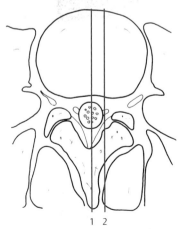

1 2

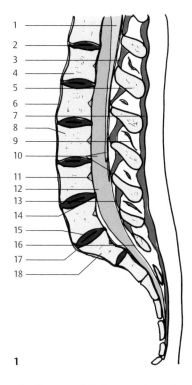
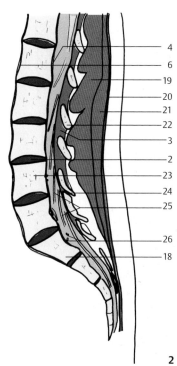

1
2

1 Conus medullaris
2 Intervertebral disk
(with "intranuclear cleft" signifying
an adult disk on MRI)
3 Ligamenta flava
4 Body of L1 vertebra and posterior
longitudinal ligament
5 Spinous process of L1
6 Anterior longitudinal ligament
7 Supraspinal ligaments
8 Body of L3 vertebra
9 Interspinal ligaments
(with interspinal bursa)
10 Cauda equina
11 Basivertebral veins
12 Thecal space

13 Dura
14 Superior vertebral end plate
15 Inferior vertebral end plate
16 Epidural fat
17 Promontory
18 Sacral vertebra (S1)
19 Multifidus muscles
20 Lumbosacral fascia
21 Erector spinae muscle
22 Vertebral arch
23 Body of L4 vertebra
24 Facet joint
25 Nerve roots
26 Internal vertebral venous
plexus

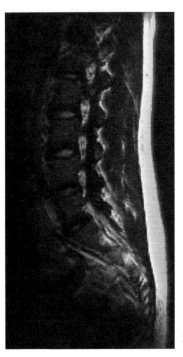
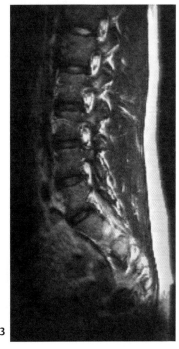

3

4

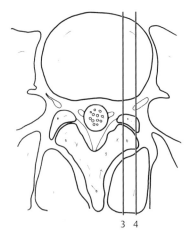

3 4

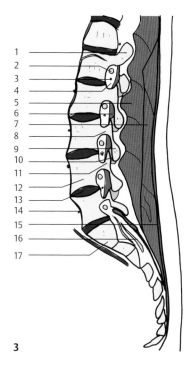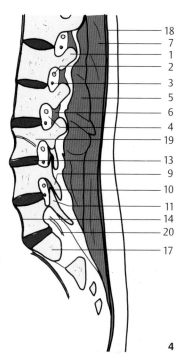

3   4

1	Mamillary process	12	Body of L4 vertebra
2	Spinal nerve L1	13	Intervertebral disk
3	Spinal branch of segmental artery	14	Anterior longitudinal ligament
4	Intervertebral foramen	15	Lumbodorsal ligament
5	Multifidus muscle	16	Sacral nerve roots
6	Ligamentum flavum	17	Sacral vertebra (S1)
7	Erector spinae muscle	18	Lumbodorsal (thoracolumbar) fascia
8	Pedicle of L3 vertebra	19	Body of L3 vertebra
9	Inferior articular process	20	Spinal nerve L5
10	Facet joint		
11	Superior articular process		

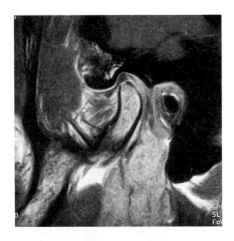

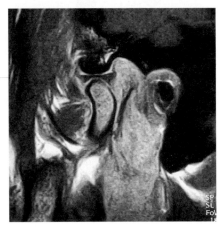

Cranial

Anterior ☐ Posterior

Caudal

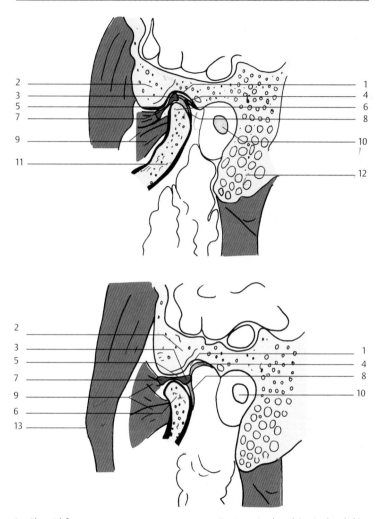

1 Glenoid fossa
2 Articular tubercle
3 Posterior band (articular disk)
4 Superior retrodiscal lamina of
   bilaminar zone
5 Intermediate (or thin) zone
   (articular disk)
6 Mandibular condyle

7 Anterior band (articular disk)
8 Posterior retrodiscal lamina of
   bilaminar zone
9 Lateral pterygoid muscle
10 External auditory canal
11 Neck of condyle
12 Mastoid
13 Temporalis muscle

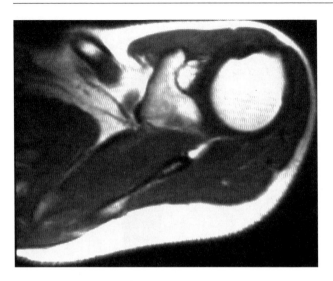

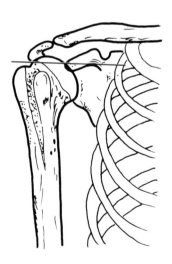

Anterior

Medial ▢ Lateral

Posterior

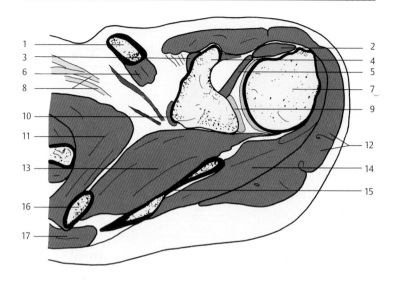

1 Clavicle
2 Supraspinatus muscle (tendon)
3 Pectoralis minor muscle (tendon)
4 Coracoid process
5 Biceps muscle (long head, tendon)
6 Subclavius muscle
7 Humeral head
8 Brachial plexus
9 Glenoid

10 Coracoclavicular ligament
11 Serratus anterior muscle
12 Deltoid muscle
13 Supraspinatus muscle
14 Infraspinatus muscle
15 Spine of scapula
16 Rib
17 Trapezius muscle

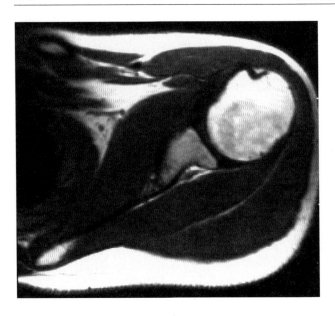

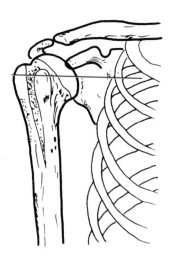

Anterior

Medial ☐ Lateral

Posterior

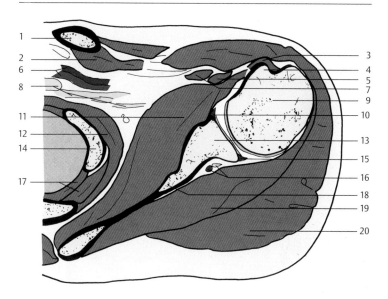

1 Clavicle
2 Subclavius muscle
3 Biceps muscle (long head, tendon)
4 Lesser tuberosity
5 Biceps brachii muscle (short head)
6 Axillary artery and vein
7 Coracobrachialis muscle
8 Brachial plexus
9 Humeral head
10 Anterior glenoid labrum
11 Subscapularis muscle

12 Serratus anterior muscle
13 Glenoid
14 Rib
15 Posterior glenoid labrum
16 Suprascapular artery, vein and nerve
17 Intercostal muscles
18 Scapula
19 Teres minor muscle
20 Deltoid muscle

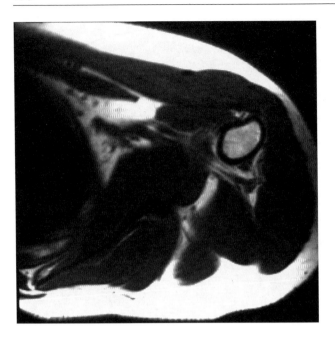

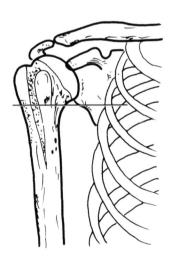

Anterior

Medial ☐ Lateral

Posterior

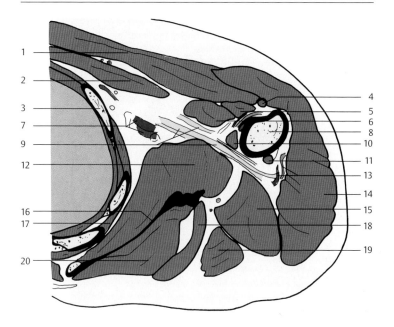

1 Pectoralis major muscle
2 Pectoralis minor muscle
3 Rib
4 Biceps brachii muscle (long head)
5 Biceps brachii muscle (short head)
6 Coracobrachialis muscle
7 Axillary artery and vein
8 Humerus
9 Brachial plexus
10 Subscapularis muscle
11 Triceps brachii muscle (lateral head)

12 Subscapularis muscle
13 Posterior circumflex humeral artery and vein
14 Deltoid muscle
15 Triceps brachii muscle (long head)
16 Scapula
17 Serratus anterior muscle
18 Teres major muscle
19 Latissimus dorsi muscle
20 Infraspinatus muscle

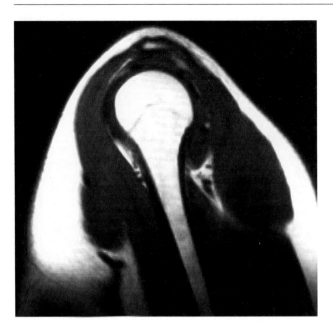

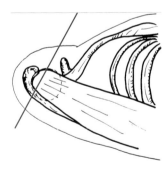

Proximal

Anterior ☐ Posterior

Distal

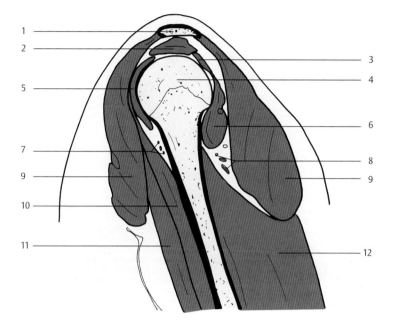

1 Acromion
2 Supraspinatus muscle (tendon)
3 Infraspinatus muscle (tendon)
4 Humeral head
5 Biceps muscle (long head, tendon)
6 Teres minor muscle
7 Anterior circumflex humeral artery and vein
8 Posterior circumflex humeral artery and vein
9 Deltoid muscle
10 Coracobrachialis muscle
11 Biceps brachii muscle (short head)
12 Triceps muscle

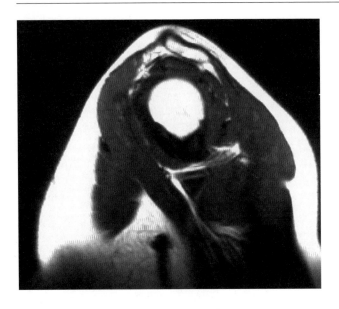

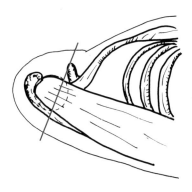

Proximal

Anterior ☐ Posterior

Distal

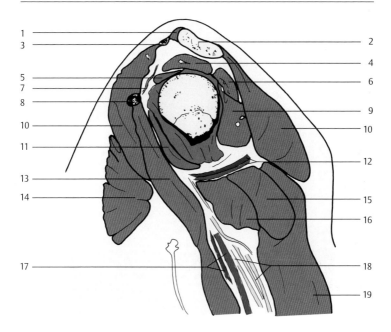

1 Trapezius muscle
2 Scapula
3 Clavicle
4 Supraspinatus muscle
5 Biceps brachii muscle (long head, tendon)
6 Intraspinatus muscle
7 Coracoacromial ligament
8 Coracoid process
9 Teres minor muscle
10 Deltoid muscle

11 Subscapularis muscle
12 Posterior circumflex humeral artery and vein
13 Coracobrachialis muscle
14 Pectoralis major muscle
15 Teres major muscle
16 Latissimus dorsi muscle
17 Brachial artery and vein
18 Brachial plexus
19 Triceps brachii muscle

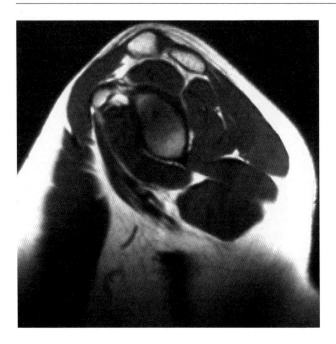

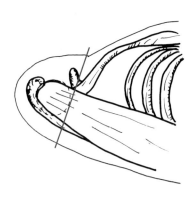

Proximal

Anterior ☐ Posterior

Distal

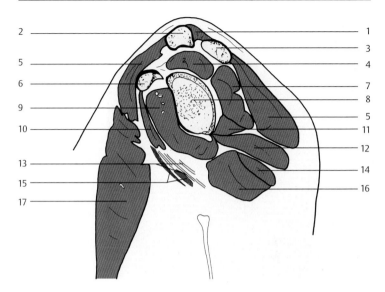

1 Trapezius muscle
2 Clavicle
3 Spine of scapula
4 Supraspinatus muscle
5 Deltoid muscle
6 Coracoid process
7 Infraspinatus muscle
8 Glenoid cavity
9 Subscapularis muscle
10 Coracobrachialis muscle
11 Teres minor muscle
12 Triceps brachii muscle
13 Brachial plexus
14 Teres major muscle
15 Axillary artery and vein
16 Latissimus dorsi muscle
17 Pectoralis major muscle

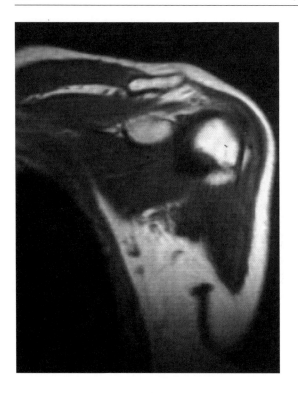

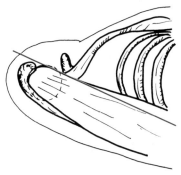

Proximal

Medial ☐ Lateral

Distal

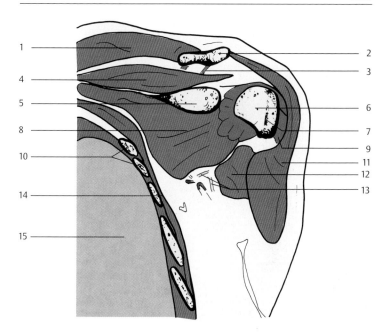

1 Trapezius muscle
2 Clavicle
3 Coracoacromial ligament
4 Supraspinatus muscle
5 Coracoid process
6 Humeral head
7 Bicipital groove
8 Subscapularis muscle

9 Articular capsule
10 Rib
11 Deltoid muscle
12 Coracobrachialis muscle
13 Brachial plexus
14 Serratus anterior muscle
15 Lung

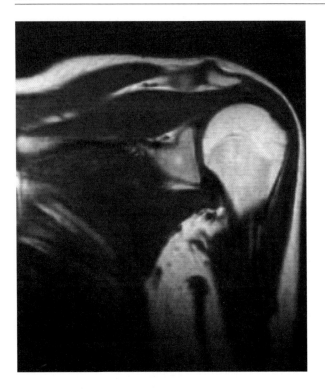

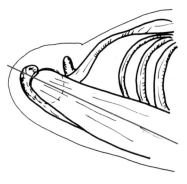

Proximal

Medial [ ] Lateral

Distal

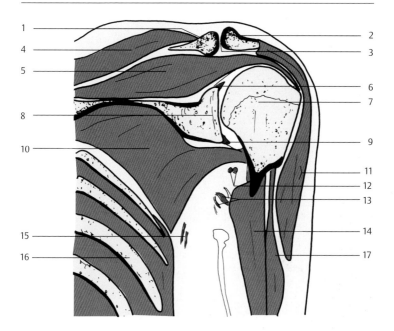

1   Clavicle
2   Acromion
3   Acromioclavicular joint
4   Trapezius muscle
5   Supraspinatus muscle (+tendon)
6   Superior glenoid labrum
7   Humeral head
8   Glenoid (scapula)
9   Inferior glenoid labrum
10 Subscapularis muscle
11 Deltoid muscle
12 Posterior circumflex humeral artery
13 Axillary artery and vein
14 Coracobrachialis muscle
15 Subscapular artery, vein and nerve
16 Ribs
17 Biceps brachii muscle (long head)

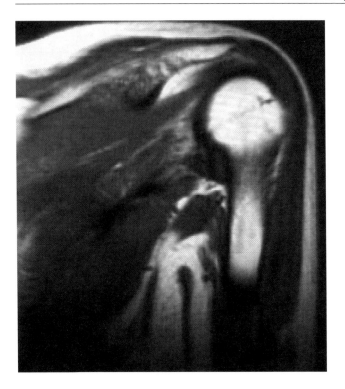

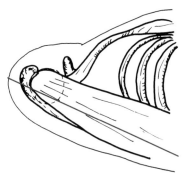

Proximal

Medial ☐ Lateral

Distal

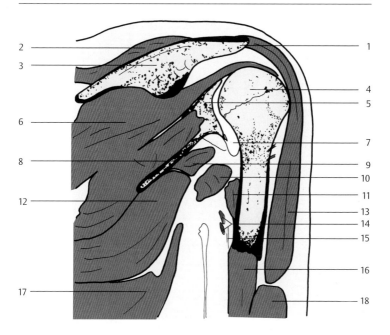

1 Acromion
2 Trapezius muscle
3 Spine of scapula
4 Humeral head
5 Glenoid
6 Infraspinatus muscle
7 Axillary recess
8 Scapula
9 Teres minor muscle
10 Latissimus dorsi muscle
11 Triceps brachii muscle
12 Teres major muscle
13 Deltoid muscle
14 Brachial artery and vein
15 Median nerve
16 Coracobrachialis muscle
17 Latissimus dorsi muscle
18 Biceps brachii muscle

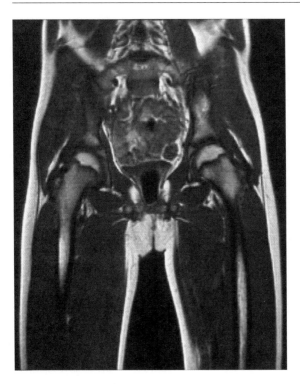

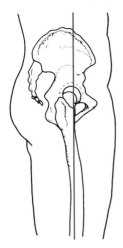

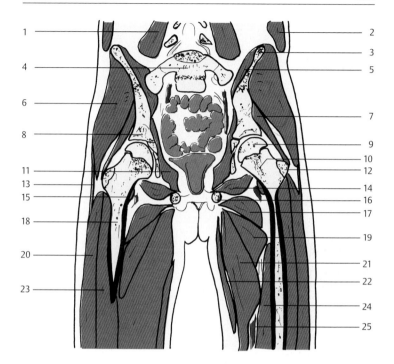

1 Psoas muscle
2 Internal oblique muscle
3 Ilium
4 Sacrum
5 Iliac muscle
6 Gluteus medius muscle
7 Gluteus minimus muscle
8 Acetabular roof (ilium)
9 Femoral head (epiphysis)
10 Femoral neck
11 Internal obturator muscle
12 Greater trochanter
13 Iliotibial tract

14 External obturator muscle
15 Iliopsoas muscle (tendon)
16 Pubis (inferior ramus)
17 Adductor brevis muscle
18 Femur
19 Adductor longus muscle
20 Vastus lateralis muscle
21 Adductor magnus muscle
22 Gracilis muscle
23 Vastus intermedius muscle
24 Vastus medialis muscle
25 Femoral artery and vein

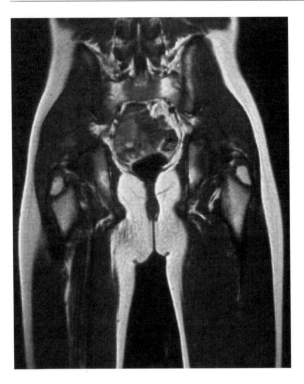

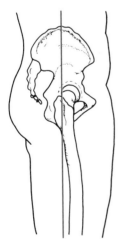

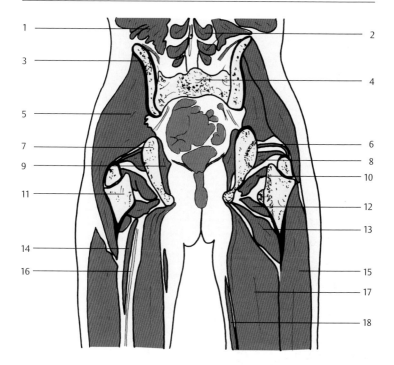

1	Quadratus lumborum muscle	**10**	Quadratus femoris muscle
2	Multifidus muscles	**11**	Femur
3	Ilium	**12**	Adductor brevis muscle
4	Sacrum	**13**	Adductor longus muscle
5	Gluteus medius muscle	**14**	Biceps femoris muscle
6	Gemellus muscles (tendon)	**15**	Vastus lateralis muscle
7	Ischium	**16**	Sciatic nerve
8	External obturator muscle	**17**	Adductor magnus muscle
9	Internal obturator muscle	**18**	Gracilis muscle

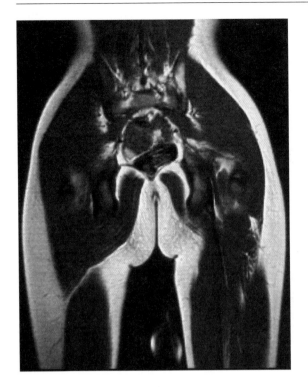

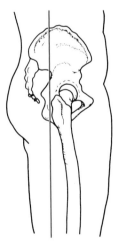

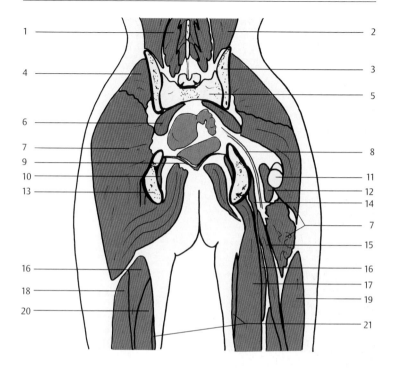

1 Multifidus muscles
2 Quadratus lumborum muscle
3 Ilium
4 Gluteus medius muscle
5 Sacrum (ala)
6 Piriform muscle
7 Gluteus maximus muscle
8 Sciatic nerve
9 Levator ani muscle
10 Internal obturator muscle
11 Greater trochanter
12 Piriform muscle
13 Ischial tuberosity
14 Semitendinosus muscle (tendon)
15 Biceps femoris muscle (long head)
16 Semitendinosus muscle
17 Abductor magnus muscle
18 Biceps femoris muscle
   (short head)
19 Vastus lateralis muscle
20 Semimembranosus muscle
21 Gracilis muscle

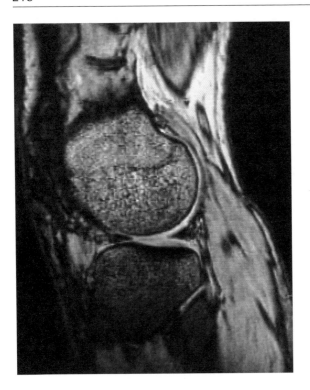

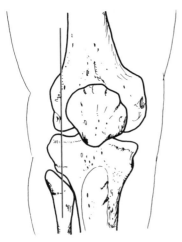

Proximal

Anterior [ ] Posterior

Distal

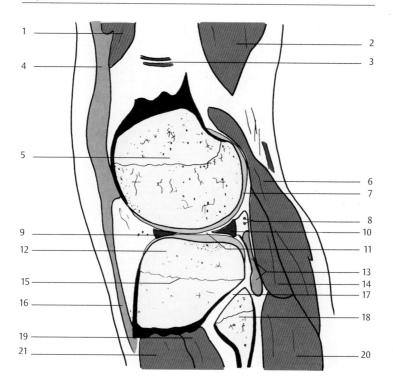

1 Vastus lateralis muscle
2 Biceps femoris muscle
3 Lateral superior genicular artery
4 Lateral patellar retinaculum
5 Lateral femoral condyle
6 Gastrocnemius muscle (lateral head)
7 Articular cartilage
8 Lateral inferior genicular artery
9 Lateral meniscus (anterior horn)
10 Lateral meniscus (posterior horn)
11 Knee joint space
12 Lateral tibial condyle
13 Popliteus muscle (tendon)
14 Plantaris muscle
15 Epiphyseal line
16 Patellar ligament
17 Tibiofibular joint
18 Fibula
19 Extensor digitorum longus muscle
20 Soleus muscle
21 Tibialis anterior muscle

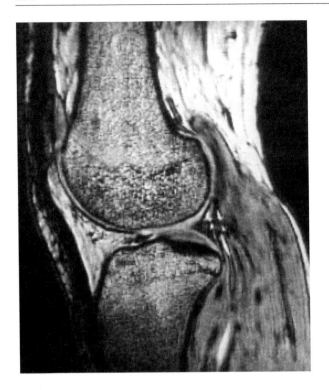

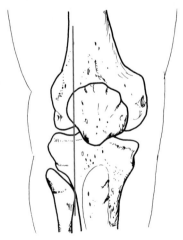

Proximal

Anterior ☐ Posterior

Distal

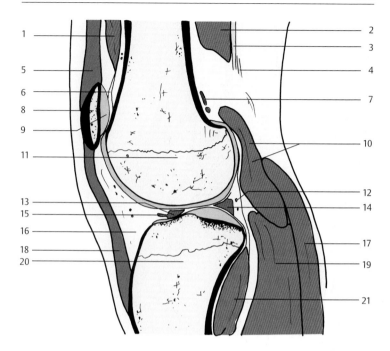

1 Vastus intermedius muscle
2 Biceps femoris muscle
3 Common peroneal nerve
4 Tibial nerve
5 Quadriceps femoris muscle (tendon)
6 Suprapatellar bursa
7 Lateral superior genicular artery
8 Patella
9 Retropatellar cartilage
10 Plantaris muscle
11 Lateral femoral condyle

12 Lateral inferior genicular artery
13 Lateral meniscus (anterior horn)
14 Lateral meniscus (posterior horn)
15 Transverse ligament of knee
16 Infrapatellar fat pad
17 Gastrocnemius muscle
   (lateral head)
18 Patellar ligament
19 Soleus muscle
20 Tibia
21 Popliteus muscle

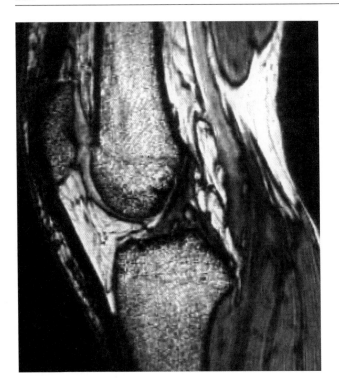

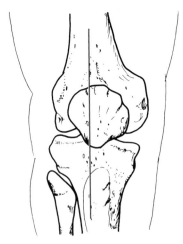

Proximal

Anterior □ Posterior

Distal

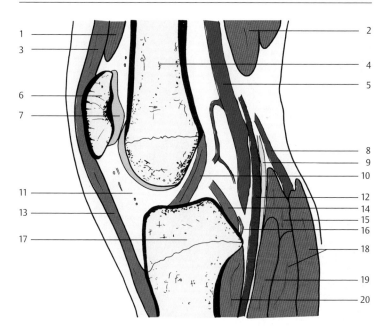

1 Vastus medialis muscle
2 Semimembranosus muscle
3 Rectus femoris muscle (tendon)
4 Femur
5 Femoral vein
6 Patella
7 Retropatellar cartilage
8 Short saphenous vein
9 Tibial nerve
10 Anterior cruciate ligament
11 Infrapatellar fat pad
12 Popliteal artery
13 Patellar ligament
14 Posterior cruciate ligament
15 Gastrocnemius muscle (medial head)
16 Posterior meniscofemoral ligament
17 Tibia
18 Gastrocnemius muscle (lateral head)
19 Soleus muscle
20 Popliteus muscle

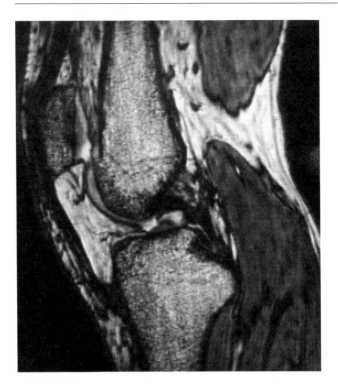

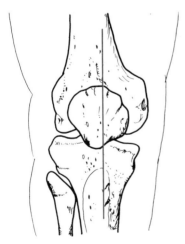

Proximal

Anterior ☐ Posterior

Distal

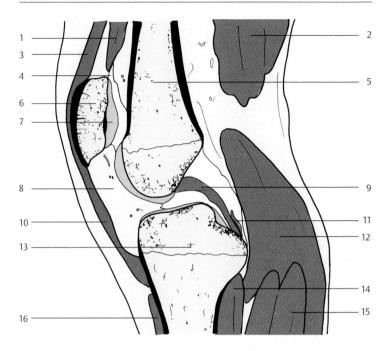

1 Vastus medialis muscle
2 Semimembranosus muscle
3 Quadriceps femoris muscle (tendon)
4 Suprapatellar bursa
5 Femur
6 Patella
7 Retropatellar cartilage
8 Infrapatellar fat pad
9 Posterior cruciate ligament
10 Patellar ligament
11 Posterior meniscofemoral ligament
12 Gastrocnemius muscle
13 Tibia
14 Popliteus muscle
15 Soleus muscle
16 Tibialis anterior muscle

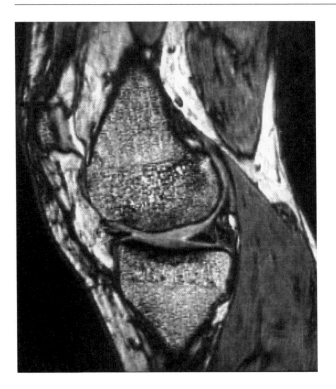

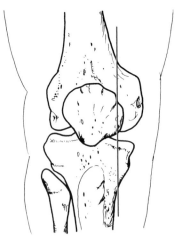

Proximal

Anterior ☐ Posterior

Distal

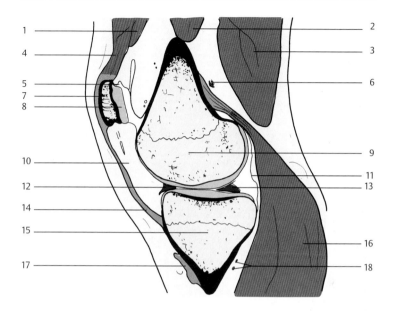

1 Vastus medialis muscle
2 Sartorius muscle
3 Semimembranosus muscle
4 Quadriceps femoris muscle
 (quadriceps tendon)
5 Suprapatellar bursa
6 Medial superior genicular artery
 and vein
7 Patella
8 Retropatellar cartilage
9 Medial femoral condyle
10 Infrapatellar fat pad

11 Joint capsule
12 Medial meniscus (anterior horn)
13 Medial meniscus (posterior horn)
14 Patellar ligament
15 Medial tibial condyle
16 Gastrocnemius muscle
 (medial head)
17 Sartorius muscle
 (tendon attachment)
18 Medial inferior genicular artery
 and vein

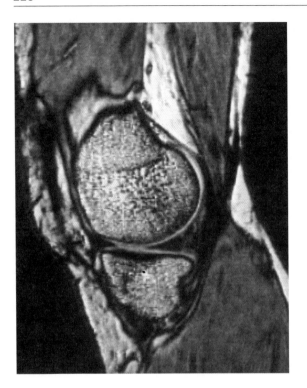

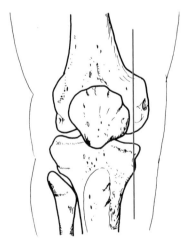

Proximal

Anterior ☐ Posterior

Distal

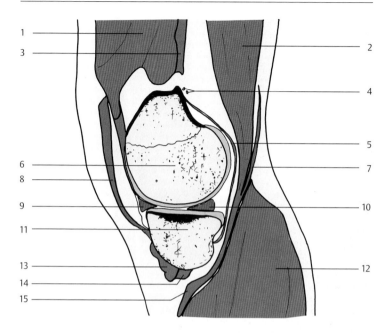

1 Vastus medialis muscle
2 Semimembranosus muscle
3 Adductor magnus muscle (tendon)
4 Medial superior genicular artery and vein
5 Joint capsule
6 Medial femoral condyle
7 Semitendinosus muscle (tendon)
8 Medial patellar retinaculum
9 Medial meniscus (anterior horn)
10 Medial meniscus (posterior horn)
11 Tibia
12 Gastrocnemius muscle (medial head)
13 Sartorius muscle (tendon attachment)
14 Gracilis muscle (tendon attachment)
15 Pes anserinus

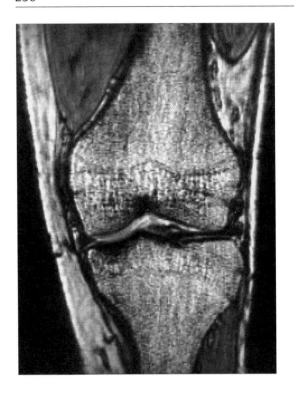

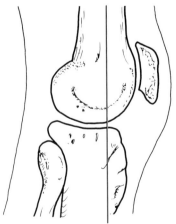

Proximal

Medial [ ] Lateral

Distal

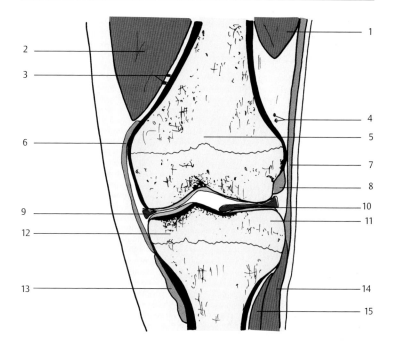

1 Vastus lateralis muscle
2 Vastus medialis muscle
3 Medial superior genicular artery
4 Lateral superior genicular artery
5 Femur
6 Medial collateral ligament
7 Iliotibial tract
8 Popliteus muscle (tendon)

9 Medial meniscus
   (intermediate part)
10 Lateral meniscus (anterior horn)
11 Lateral tibial plateau
12 Medial tibial plateau
13 Pes anserinus
14 Peroneus longus muscle
15 Extensor digitorum longus muscle

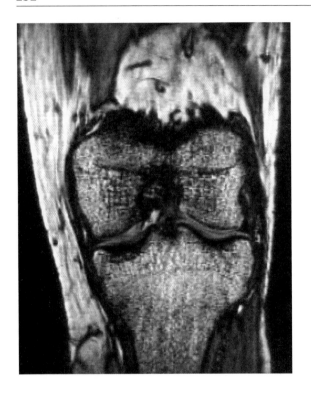

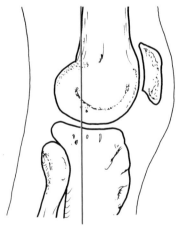

Proximal

Medial   Lateral

Distal

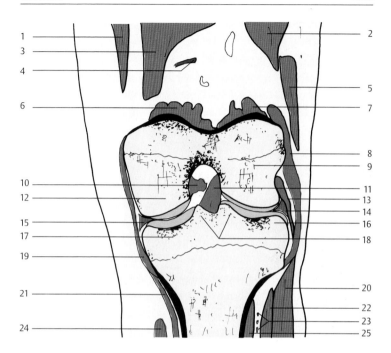

1 Sartorius muscle
2 Vastus lateralis muscle
3 Semimembranosus muscle
4 Medial superior genicular artery
5 Biceps femoris muscle
6 Gastrocnemius muscle
(medial head)
7 Gastrocnemius muscle
(lateral head)
8 Iliotibial tract
9 Lateral femoral condyle
10 Posterior cruciate ligament
11 Anterior cruciate ligament
12 Medial femoral condyle
13 Popliteus muscle (tendon)

14 Lateral meniscus (intermediate
part)
15 Medial meniscus
(intermediate part)
16 Lateral tibial plateau
17 Medial tibial plateau
18 Intercondylar eminence
19 Medial collateral ligament
20 Peroneus longus muscle
21 Gracilis muscle (tendon)
22 Extensor digitorum longus muscle
23 Lateral inferior genicular artery
and vein
24 Semitendinosus muscle (tendon)
25 Tibialis posterior muscle

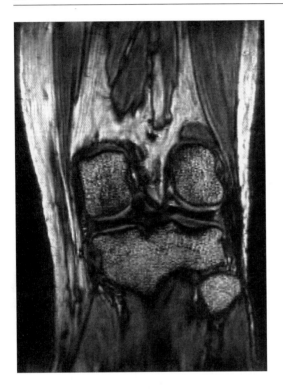

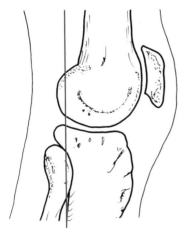

Proximal

Medial ☐ Lateral

Distal

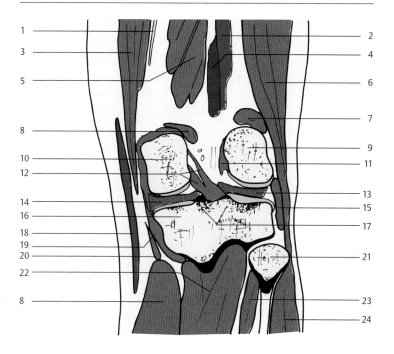

1 Saphenous nerve
2 Popliteal vein
3 Sartorius muscle
4 Popliteal artery
5 Semimembranosus muscle
6 Biceps femoris muscle
7 Gastrocnemius muscle (lateral head)
8 Gastrocnemius muscle (medial head)
9 Lateral femoral condyle
10 Medial femoral condyle
11 Anterior cruciate ligament
12 Posterior cruciate ligament
13 Lateral meniscus (intermediate part)

14 Medial meniscus
(intermediate part)
15 Popliteus muscle (tendon)
16 Medial tibial condyle
17 Intercondylar eminence
18 Long saphenous vein
19 Semimembranosus muscle
(tendon)
20 Gracilis muscle (tendon)
21 Head of fibula
22 Popliteus muscle
23 Tibialis posterior muscle
24 Peroneus longus muscle

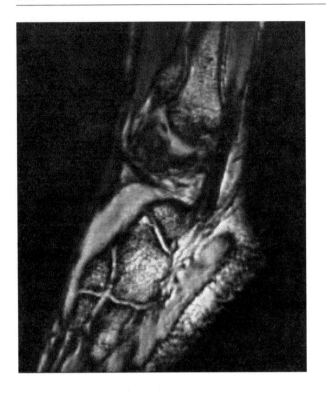

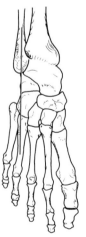

Proximal
Dorsal

Anterior ☐ Posterior

Plantar
Distal

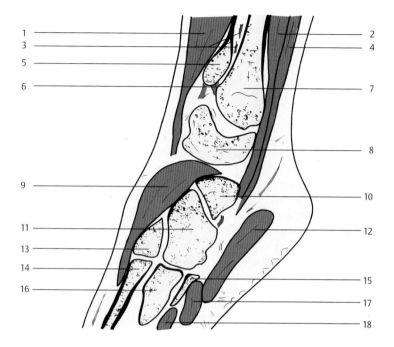

1 Extensor digitorum longus muscle
2 Peroneus longus muscle
3 Anterior tibial artery and vein
4 Peroneus brevis muscle
5 Tibia
6 Anterior tibiofibular ligament
7 Fibula (lateral malleolus)
8 Talus
9 Extensor digitorum brevis muscle

10 Calcaneus
11 Cuboid bone
12 Abductor digiti minimi muscle
13 Lateral cuneiform bone
14 Third metatarsal bone
15 Fifth metatarsal bone
16 Fourth metatarsal bone
17 Flexor digiti minimi muscle
18 Interosseous muscle

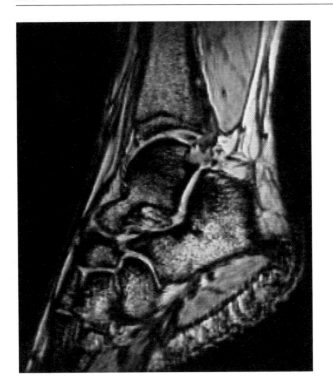

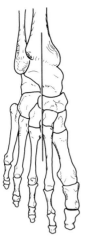

Proximal
Dorsal

Anterior ☐ Posterior

Plantar
Distal

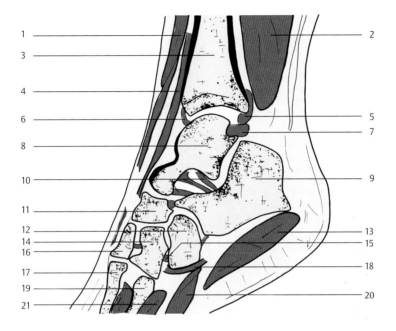

1 Extensor hallucis longus muscle	**12** Cuboid bone
2 Flexor hallucis longus muscle	**13** Abductor digiti minimi muscle
3 Tibia	**14** Lateral cuneiform bone
4 Extensor digitorum longus muscle (tendon)	**15** Interosseous ligament
	16 Intermediate cuneiform bone
5 Posterior tibiofibular ligament	**17** Second metatarsal bone
6 Joint capsule	**18** Peroneus longus muscle (tendon)
7 Posterior talofibular ligament	**19** Third metatarsal bone
8 Talus	**20** Opponens digiti minimi muscle
9 Calcaneus	**21** Lumbrical and interosseous muscles
10 Interosseous talocalcaneal ligament	
11 Navicular bone	

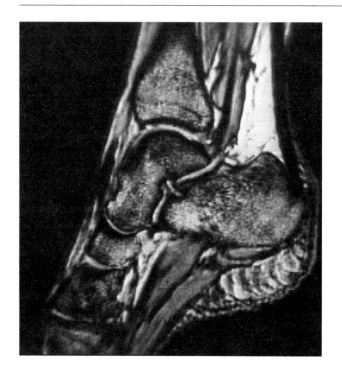

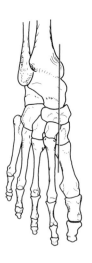

Proximal
Dorsal

Anterior ☐ Posterior

Plantar
Distal

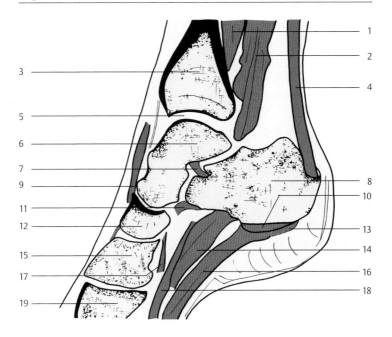

1 Tibialis posterior muscle	**11** Plantar calcaneonavicular
2 Flexor hallucis longus muscle	ligament
3 Tibia	**12** Navicular bone
4 Achilles tendon	**13** Plantar aponeurosis
5 Talocrural joint (tibiotalar part)	**14** Quadratus plantae muscle
6 Talus	**15** Intermediate cuneiform bone
7 Interosseous talocalcaneal	**16** Flexor digitorum brevis muscle
ligament	**17** Tibialis posterior muscle (tendon)
8 Calcaneus	**18** Flexor digitorum longus muscle
9 Tibialis anterior muscle (tendon)	(tendon)
10 Abductor digiti minimi muscle	**19** Second metatarsal bone (base)

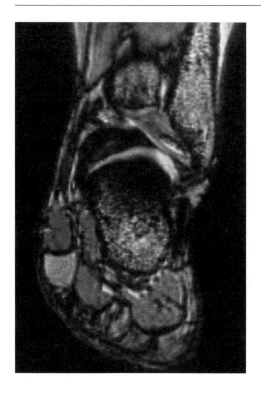

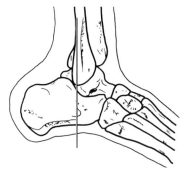

Proximal

Medial ☐ Lateral

Distal

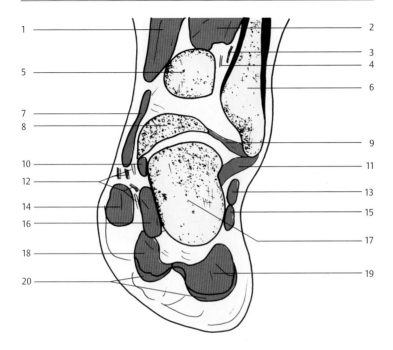

1 Tibialis posterior muscle
2 Flexor hallucis longus muscle
3 Anterior tibial artery
4 Deep peroneal nerve
5 Tibia
6 Fibula
7 Flexor digitorum longus muscle (tendon)
8 Talus
9 Posterior talofibular ligament
10 Flexor hallucis longus muscle (tendon)

11 Calcaneofibular ligament
12 Medial and lateral plantar artery, vein and nerve
13 Peroneus brevis muscle (tendon)
14 Abductor hallucis muscle
15 Peroneus longus muscle (tendon)
16 Quadratus plantae muscle
17 Calcaneus
18 Flexor digitorum brevis muscle
19 Abductor digiti minimi muscle
20 Plantar aponeurosis

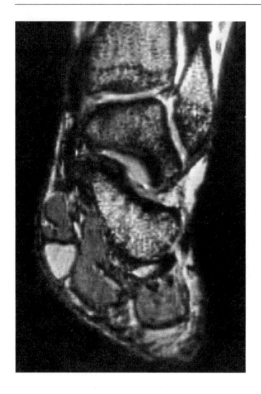

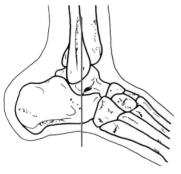

Proximal

Medial ☐ Lateral

Distal

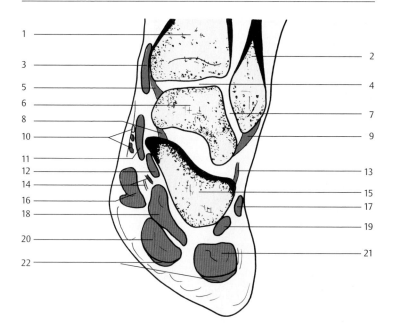

1 Tibia
2 Fibula
3 Tibialis posterior muscle (tendon)
4 Talocrural joint (tibiotalar part)
5 Deltoid ligament
(posterior tibiotalar part)
6 Talus
7 Talocrural joint (fibulotalar part)
8 Interosseous talocalcaneal ligament
9 Posterior talofibular ligament
10 Medial plantar artery, vein
and nerve
11 Flexor digitorum longus muscle
(tendon)

12 Flexor hallucis longus muscle
(tendon)
13 Calcaneofibular ligament
14 Lateral plantar artery, vein and
nerve
15 Calcaneus
16 Abductor hallucis muscle
17 Peroneus brevis muscle (tendon)
18 Quadratus plantae muscle
19 Peroneus longus muscle (tendon)
20 Flexor digitorum brevis muscle
21 Abductor digiti minimi muscle
22 Plantar aponeurosis

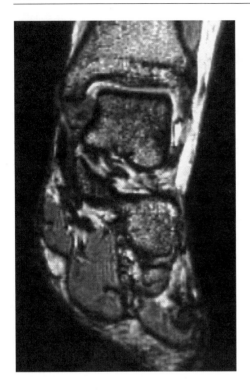

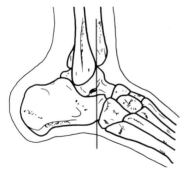

Proximal

Medial ☐ Lateral

Distal

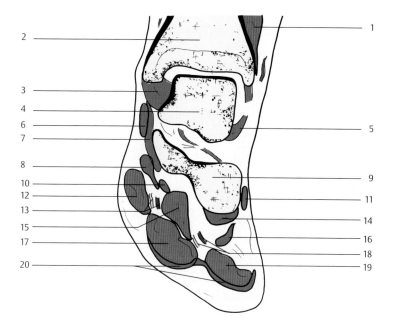

1 Extensor digitorum longus muscle
2 Tibia
3 Deltoid ligament
(posterior tibiotalar part)
4 Talus
5 Anterior talofibular ligament
6 Tibialis posterior muscle (tendon)
7 Deltoid ligament
(tibiocalcaneal part)
8 Flexor digitorum longus muscle
(tendon)
9 Calcaneus
10 Flexor hallucis longus muscle
(tendon)

11 Peroneus brevis muscle (tendon)
12 Abductor hallucis muscle
13 Medial plantar artery, vein and
nerve
14 Long plantar ligament
15 Quadratus plantae muscle
16 Peroneus longus muscle (tendon)
17 Flexor digitorum brevis muscle
18 Lateral plantar artery, vein and
nerve
19 Abductor digiti minimi muscle
20 Plantar aponeurosis

References

Basset, L. W., R. H. Gold, L. L. Seeger: MRI Atlas of the Musculoskelettal System. Deutscher Ärzte-Verlag, Köln 1989.

Beyer-Enke, S. A., K. Tiedemann, J. Görich, A. Gamroth: Dünnschichtcomputertomographie der Schädelbasis, Radiologe 27 1987: 438–488

Cahill, D. R., M. J. Orland, C. C. Reading: Atlas of Human Cross-Sectional Anatomy. Wiley-Liss 1990

Chacko, A. K., R. W. Katzberg, A. Mac Kay: MRI Atlas of Normal Anatomy. McGraw-Hill Inc., New York 1991

El-Khoury, G. Y., R. A. Bergman, E. J. Montgomery: Sectional Anatomy by MRI/CT. Churchill, Livingstone 1990

Feneis, H.: Pocket Atlas of Human Anatomy, Thieme, Stuttgart 1994

Han-Kim: Sectional Human Anatomy. Ilchokak, Seoul; Igaku-Shoin, New York-Tokyo 1989

Huk, W. J., G. Gademann, G. Freidmann: MRI of Central Nervous System Diseases. Springer, Berlin 1990

Kahle, W., H. Leonhard, W. Platzer: Pocket Atlas of Anatomie. Thieme, Stuttgart 1993

Kang, M. S., D. Resnick: MRI of the Extremities: An Anatomic Atlas. W. B. Saunders Company, Philadelphia 1991

Koritke, J. G., H. Sick: Atlas of Sectional Human Anatomy. Urban & Schwarzenberg, Baltimore – München 1988

Kretschmann, H.-J., W. Weinrich: Klinische Neuroanatomie und kranielle Bilddiagnostik, Thieme, Stuttgart 1991

Leblanc, A.: Anatomy and Imaging of the Cranial Nerves, Springer, Berlin 1992

Meschan, I.: Synopsis of Radiologic Anatomy. W. B. Saunders Company, Philadelphia

Middleton, W. D., T. L. Lawson (eds.): Anatomy and MRI of the Joints. Raven Press 1989

Möller, T. B., E. Reif: MR-Atlas des muskuloskelettalen Systems. Blackwell, Berlin 1993

Rauber/Kopsch: Anatomie des Menschen. Lehrbuch und Atlas (Hrsg. H. Leonhardt, B. Tillmann, G. Töndury, K. Zilles). Band I Bewegungsapparat. Thieme, Stuttgart 1987

Richter, E., T. Feyerabend: Normal Lymph Node Topography. Springer, Berlin 1991

Schnitzlein, H. N., F. Reed Murtagh: Imaging Atlas of the Head and Spine. Urban & Schwarzenberg, Baltimore 1990

Stark, D. D., W. G. Bradley: Magnetic Resonance Imaging. Mosby, St. Louis 1999

v. Hagens, G., L. J. Romrell, M. H. Ross, K. Tiedemann: The Visible Human Body. Lea & Febinger, Philadelphia 1991

Wegener, O. H.: Ganzkörpercomputertomographie. Blackwell, Berlin 1992

Witzig, H.: Punkt-Punkt-Komma-Strich. Falken Niedernhausen 1991

Index

W